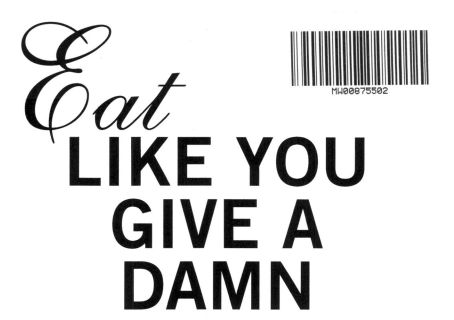

Eat LIKE YOU GIVE A DAMN

*Give Up, Give In, or Give it
All You've Got!*

JUDY MOLINARO

ISBN-10: 1517372232
ISBN-13: 978-1517372231

For bulk rate discounts contact:
judy@judymolinaro.com or 386.871.0582

Visit Judy at:
www.judymolinaro.com
www.facebook.com/fityouwellness

Cover Design by Pam Carrier

Cover Photo by Paul Vicario
www.vicariostudio.com

Interior and eBook Design by Tru Publishing
www.trupublishing.com

This book is dedicated to you.

Now is the time to envision a healthier life for you.
Today is the day to commit, to take action, and to make changes.
You've got this!

Your success will be intentional, not accidental.
Move forward knowing you are in charge.

Judy Molinaro

Contents

Foreword

Judy Molinaro's book, Eat Like You Give a Damn, is a refreshing and much-needed book for anyone trying to navigate their way through the vast number of self-help and wellness books available on the market today. Too many people trying to implement a wellness plan get bogged down and lost in the morass of misinformation, fluff, and pure nonsense that permeates the fitness and wellness industry. The reality is that it's not quite that complicated, and Judy's book spells it out step-by-step for someone who is more interested in results than research. Her 3 R approach is spot on, effective, easy to understand, and practical-because it works, pure and simple.

In an age where few people take personal responsibility for their lives and the results they get from anything, her personal responsibility approach is the only sure way to guarantee that you will get the results that you are seeking. Judy stresses that you and you alone, are responsible for your health and wellness. She explains, step-by-step in a how-to-format what you need to do in order to get your mind and body moving in the right direction. Unlike a lot of diet and fitness gurus, she's acutely aware that it starts with you, and your mental strength and willpower. If you follow her advice, willpower and the results you desire, will surely follow.

There are a lot of more complicated diet and wellness books out there on the market that you could read and, if you want an exercise in futility, they are there for you. If you want results, you hold the answer right in your hands, right now. Follow her advice, use this book, and start feeling better about yourself, your body, and your life. Make a decision, make an excuse or make progress. After opening this book, the choice is yours.

—John Sannicandro

John Sannicandro has been a teacher, psychotherapist, athletic coach, author, and personal coach for over 30 years. He is a Licensed Mental Health Counselor, Certified Mind Body Coach, Certified Life Coach, and a Certified Hypnotherapist. He has been an athlete and fitness enthusiast his entire life and is an avid martial artist practicing Uechi Ryu Karate for the past 25 years. His unique qualifications and passion make him the ideal coach for those seeking to take their life, health, and wellness to the next level. You can contact him at mindbodycoach.org, where he also writes weekly on self-help, personal development, and mind body coaching.

A journey of a thousand miles begins with a single step.
Lao-Tzu

Introduction

Take Ownership of Your Choices

We must stop digging our graves with forks and spoons!
Judy Molinaro

While getting older is unavoidable, do you feel as if you are falling apart along the way? Daily self-care is paramount to living an abundant, vibrant, and fulfilling way of life. Recognizing that diets don't work and lifestyles do, Eat Like You Give A Damn addresses the need of lifestyle management and focuses on simple, easy to learn and incorporate daily habits to improve mind, diet, and exercise for peak health, wellness, and productivity. A balanced diet and exercise not only changes your body, it changes your mind, your attitude, and your mood. Food is the most abused anxiety drug and exercise is the most underutilized antidepressant.

As a health and wellness speaker, yoga instructor, and fitness consultant, I regularly address people who have neglected their physical and mental well-being and want to learn more about living a stronger and more energetic lifestyle. They are suffering from common social ills related to issues such as work and media overload, money and economy concerns, family responsibilities, and relationship issues. The consequences of these struggles result in a health crisis; often times poor nutrition, obesity, extreme stress, sleep deprivation and the like are robbing them of experiencing optimal vitality.

Being overweight has become the norm, but it is not normal. Almost two-thirds of all Americans need to lose weight and the number is growing at an alarming rate. The Centers for Disease Control report that the US is the world's most obese major country and it has reached an all-time high. Nearly 40% of adult men and women aged 40 to 64 are obese and close behind at 30% are 20 to 39 year olds. A Harvard School of Public Health study reports the nation spends an estimated $190 billion a year treating obesity related conditions. Obesity and lack of exercise are responsible for approximately 1,000 American deaths each day and if the trend continues they will soon overtake smoking as the leading preventable cause of death in the US.

The American Psychological Association reports that 77% of people in the US regularly experience symptoms caused by stress. High and constant stress levels can negatively affect a person's physical and mental health and not everyone is coping well. Job stress is estimated to cost US industry more than $300 billion a year in absenteeism, turnover, diminished productivity, and medical, legal and insurance costs. Over 60% of people surveyed say it is extremely important to manage stress, eat a healthy diet, and be physically active, yet they have a hard time accomplishing these goals.

Eat Like You Give A Damn encourages you to take responsibility for your actions. What you put in your mouth, how active you are, and the thoughts that you think are well within your control. You have free will which means that you are completely responsible for all of your successes and failures. When you are responsible for every action you take and every decision you make, there is virtually nothing that you cannot achieve; taking responsibility for your actions equals success. It's only when you accept that everything you are or ever will be is up to you; it's only then that you can lead yourself in the direction needed to shape the outcome of your wellness goals.

To get the most from this book read it in order from front to back; each chapter's lessons teach and build upon the next. It has been structured into categories; The Three R's, Right Mind, Right Food, and Right Exercise. It's further broken down into subheadings so you won't waste time flipping through pages to find the information needed to refresh your memory.

For your convenience I have designed a free companion workbook so you can easily answer questions and make notes. Download and print it at www.judymolinaro.com/p/workbook.

There are no points to count and no meetings to attend. An everyday spiral bound notebook is all that's required to keep track of your dietary intake, level of activity, and day to day happenings. Keeping a daily log will be of use in identifying your positive and negative eating habits and exercise patterns. As well, it will require you to take ownership of your mistakes and responsibility for your actions so that you are accountable for your results. More people would learn from their mistakes if they weren't so busy denying them.

Stop focusing solely on losing weight and ditch the negative self-talk; being healthy should not be your destination it should be your way of life. Instead, use the straightforward system in this book to set your sights on forming and instituting a sound dietary and exercise routine; be a product of your decisions, not of your circumstances. By introducing basic daily dietary strategies and easy to implement activities these practices will help you start simple and put you on the path to regain and maintain your health. One of the greatest gifts you can give your family and loved ones is a healthy you.

If you begin right now you will start seeing the results one day earlier than if you wait until tomorrow. So take the first step today. No more waiting until Monday, the first of the month, or whatever excuse you have to put off until tomorrow what you can begin to do today. The smallest step in the right direction will end up being the biggest step of your life. Tip toe if you must but at least take the step. You cannot wait until everything is just right because it never will be. There will always be demands, hurdles, and less than perfect conditions. So what? Get started now. Once you start to see the results the energy begins to flow and you will become the most positive and determined person you know.

Finally, beware of the naysayers! There are so many people that don't care, don't want to see you succeed and who will tell you that you can't. What you've got to do is turn around and say "Watch me". Because 30 days from now you're either going to be blown away by how much you've improved in how you look, feel, and perform or you're going to regret not having done your best. The choice is yours.

THE THREE R'S

Right Mind

Minute by minute, thought by thought, your mind shapes your life.
Gurumayi

Are you really hungry? Are you feeding your body or are you feeding your emotions? Your brain can make recognizing what you need as opposed to what you want very hard to understand. Our relationship with food often changes; when you're feeling unhappy, stressed out, excited, lonely, or bored, you may try to fix those feelings with food. So before you eat, it's important to stop and think; clarify if it's your stomach that is hungry or if it's your mind and heart that needs attention instead. If you're eating for any reason besides physical hunger, you need to reconsider it. The foundation of your success will be identifying your emotions versus your physical needs and practicing a few simple principles every day.

EMOTIONAL HUNGER OR PHYSICAL HUNGER?

Do you know the difference between emotional hunger and physical hunger? While the signs may seem identical there are a number of traits that distinguish emotional hunger from physical hunger. Learning their unique characteristics will enable you to take charge of your eating habits; this knowledge and awareness will assist you in preventing emotional eating episodes.

Emotional hunger comes on fast and is in reaction to your feelings; it's not about the food but it's the only thing on your mind. If you're inclined to eat for emotional reasons any feeling that is difficult to process may trigger the urge to eat. For example, you may feel sad and turn to food for relief, or you may feel excited and react by eating. Recognize that it's not the feeling itself that sparks the impulse to eat; it's the failure to let the feeling be present without desensitizing it with food.

Physical hunger builds a little at a time and comes about because your body needs energy; it is biologically based and connected to your blood sugar levels. If you're tuned into your body you may notice cues; a growling stomach, feeling grouchy, the inability to think well or focus, fatigue, or a headache. Food is something you wish for, but it can wait.

Emotional hunger is unrelated to the time since your last meal and you will notice that you crave specific foods like ice cream, potato chips, or cookies. Emotional eating episodes are a vicious cycle. You eat because you want to feel better, and initially you feel better because food numbs your feelings, then guilt replaces the feelings that triggered the compulsion to eat in the first place. The cycle continues and your hunger persists despite fullness.

Physical hunger occurs several hours after a meal and you're open to many good choices. Foods like fruits and vegetables are appealing to your grumbling stomach; because you are satisfied you can make a conscious choice to stop eating by responding to the sensation of fullness. Eating to quell physical hunger fulfills a necessary need and there is no guilt because you know eating nourishes your body.

If you battle with emotional eating, understand it's not about finding the right nutritional plan. It's about identifying your problems and directing your strength and desire for health and wellness toward solutions. Ask yourself "What do I feel?" and "What do I need to do to feel better?" Engage in healthy pastimes before you choose to eat due to emotional hunger. Burn some energy by being active, take a walk or exercise, try something relaxing like reading or taking a bath, practice yoga and breathing exercises.

You will feel better when you take the steps necessary to help you acknowledge and handle your feelings. Keep in mind, if you change the way you look at things, the things you look at will change. It's imperative to remove anger, regret, resentment, guilt, blame, and worry; then watch your health and life improve.

What emotions and events trigger you to eat?

Why is this happening? Is there a pattern? (Stress at work, caring for an elderly parent, financial concerns, relationship issues, etc.)

Are there specific foods or drinks you choose to desensitize your feelings? What are they?

What can you do to be prepared for when these experiences arise ensuring that you will make healthier choices?

THE BEGINNING IS ALWAYS TODAY

Our body is a direct reflection of what's going on in our mind. Studies have shown that people who struggle throughout the day have a critical first hour beginning when they wake up. How you start your morning will impact your entire day, so it's essential to get going on the right foot.

It's important to focus on things you are grateful for because what you focus on becomes your reality. By improving your morning routine you can be more productive throughout the day. When you feel good about yourself and believe you're worth your own effort leading a healthy lifestyle becomes much easier.

A morning ritual that includes some type of exercise is the best way to jumpstart your day. For some it will be a full workout or an exercise DVD, for others 15 minutes of yoga or simply getting outside for a walk. Whatever you choose it should be practical and efficient so that you are likely to make it a habit.

What is your usual morning routine? Do you hit the snooze button over and over or do you take a few minutes to reflect and set the tone for the day? What is the first thing you say to yourself when you wake up? Go beyond thinking something is a good idea and implement it into your life. Don't chase after perfect, chase after perfectly healthy.

How do you typically start your day?

What changes could you make to begin on a more positive note?

ACCEPT RESPONSIBILITY

We all have countless opportunities to head down one path or another. Make good use of these opportunities, listen to your intuition, and be aware of the consequences if you don't. Nothing outside you stops you, you stop you and this can be a challenging perspective to accept. You can either suffer the pain of discipline or the pain of regret.

No one decides how you think, how you eat, or how much you exercise except you. Assigning blame serves no purpose; own your choices. If you have struggled and failed to eat healthier and exercise, ask yourself where you went wrong. I'm reasonably certain that you know. Be accountable and take the steps needed to solve your problems; this action is empowering and will lead to the results you are searching for.

Nearly four decades in the fitness industry has presented me with many occasions to work one on one with clients towards achieving their goals. Time and time again I have heard "I'd give anything to look like that". Really? You would give anything? Then why aren't you doing it? It's not long into the conversation that the excuses for why "anything" is no longer possible begin. The most common can be classified as the "Terrible Too's"; too busy, too tired, too hard, too early, etc. Your future is wide open and you are about to create it by what you chose to do.

Stop wearing your "busy-ness" like a badge of honor. Stop feeling obligated to be reachable 24/7 by people that have a warped sense of urgency. Stop being hijacked by the needs and desires of others. If you really want something you will find a way, if you don't you'll find an excuse.

Ask yourself how much time you spend on Facebook, LinkedIn, Instagram, and Pinterest; how often you're text messaging, emailing, and surfing the web. I challenge you to keep track of these time bandits and then convince me you don't have a half hour to devote to exercise, cook a healthy meal, or pack a nutritious lunch. Prove to me and to yourself that it's your job, your parents, your kids or whatever excuse it is that you have that's keeping you from doing what's necessary to succeed. The outcome of your day has an infinite number of possibilities. You know who is responsible for the outcome? You.

I realize that you're bombarded, overwhelmed, and have endless lists of things to do. The pressure mounts for all of us; you're no different than anyone else. Get over yourself. Start accepting responsibility for your actions, your behaviors, your decisions. You're the one who settled, you're the one that determined your path, you chose the road; you can either stay on it or get off at the next exit. It's all fun and games until your jeans don't fit.

Make a list of your possible time bandits.

Keep track of and record the amount of time you spend on them without any thought each day; my guess is you will be surprised by how much time you are devoting to them.

SELF-TALK

As you go about your daily life you are continually considering and analyzing the circumstances you find yourself in. You have an inner voice that psychologist's call 'self-talk' that determines how you comprehend every situation. Self-talk isn't just mindless chatter; it is the endless stream of unspoken thoughts that run through your head at any given moment throughout the day. These thoughts can be positive or negative and arise from logic and reason, or misconceptions and a lack of information.

If your thoughts are skewed towards the negative, self-talk has the potential to be like a runaway freight train creating its own troublesome reality. It's important to pay close attention to the things you tell yourself; recognize that your way of thinking might be self-defeating and getting in the way of achieving your goals.

Negative self-talk will influence how you live your life and keep you from getting the best out of it. Continuing to tell yourself that you can't do something can make it come true. Conquer your negative self-talk by asking yourself, "Is this way of thinking helping me to reach my goals?"

Positive self-talk allows you to approach life's difficulties in a more confident and productive way. It doesn't mean that you keep your head buried in the sand and disregard unpleasant circumstances, it means you think the best is going to come about, not the worst. A positive frame of mind enables you to cope with stressful situations and live a vibrant and energetic life. Studies indicate that optimistic people practice healthier habits and are more likely to be physically active and follow a wholesome diet.

Like food is to the body, self-talk is to the mind. Don't let junk thoughts echo in your head; stop focusing on what could go wrong and focus on what could go right. With practice your self-talk will contain less self-criticism and more self-acceptance; if your compassion doesn't include yourself it is incomplete.

POSITIVE THINKING PUT INTO PRACTICE

NEGATIVE THOUGHT	POSITIVE THOUGHT
I'll never be able to do this.	I can make this work.
I'm too out of shape.	I will start from where I'm at.
It's too hard.	I like a challenge and will do my best.
I don't know how.	I have the ability to learn new new concepts.
I don't have the time.	I will make the time because I am important.

Make a list of your negative self-talk thoughts.

Re-write them as positive self-talk thoughts.

THE UGLY TRUTH

According to the Centers for Disease Control and Prevention the average American woman weighs 166.2 pounds; almost exactly what the average American man weighed in the early 1960's. The average American man hasn't fared any better and now weighs nearly 30 pounds more at 195.5 pounds.

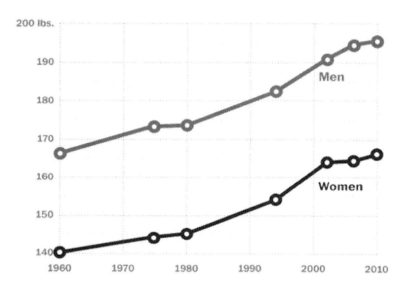

While both sexes have gained nearly an inch in height which accounts for a small amount of the weight gain it's the growing girth that is of concern. We are eating less healthy food, eating more of it and not moving as much as necessary to maintain a healthy weight. Americans are the world's third heaviest people behind the Pacific Island nations of Tonga and Micronesia. The average American is 33 pounds heavier than the average Frenchman and 40 pounds heavier than the average Japanese citizen.

Although the statistics are alarming your present situation does not need to be your final destination. It's easy to get overwhelmed and discouraged when you begin to consider lifestyle changes and accomplishing big goals. Your own self-doubt will kill more ambitions and dreams than failure ever will.

If you are committed to losing weight and regaining your overall health, wellness, and stamina you must stop focusing on dieting and start focusing on eating well and incorporating exercise into your daily life. There is one very simple way to determine what's going to happen next; be the one who makes it happen. Remember, you are in control and you have choices; give up, give in, or give it all you've got!

GOALS

Defining your goals is essential to establishing sound and clear-cut motivational strategies to reach your health and wellness intentions. However, you can't just talk about it; you've got to be about it. Your motivation will get you started, habit will keep you going, and discipline will bridge the gap between your goals and accomplishment. Look at your goals as stepping stones rather than final destinations; reaching the goal is not the end, but the means to another goal.

A goal must be well defined. Vague statements such as "I want to be thinner" or "I want to lose weight" are ambiguous. Instead determine and target your optimal weight with your physician and aim for it.

Put your goal in writing. Hectic lifestyles have a way of turning the best laid plans into distant memories. Write your goals down and keep them in a place where you will see them regularly.

State your goals with positive affirmations. An affirmation is a simply worded positive statement asserting something to be true. The affirmation "I will walk every day for a half hour, and eat fresh, healthy foods in smaller portions" is a confident and clear-cut declaration to a healthy new you!

Your goal must have a deadline for completion. To remain enthusiastic about a goal there must be an expected time of accomplishment; without it there is a lack of urgency and motivation can fade. If unexpected circumstances arise change the plan not the goal.

Goals should have a genuine emotional appeal; establish why it is important to you. Learn to prioritize your most important goals and objectives based on your sense of desire and passion.

Make your goals difficult yet realistic. Set goals in such a way that with continuous and diligent effort, you can bring them to fruition. If "Plan A" isn't working stay cool, the alphabet has 25 more letters!

State your goals in the form of a positive affirmation.

When is the expected date of accomplishment?

Why are these goals important to you?

STRIVE FOR CONSISTENCY

Every accomplishment begins with a decision to try. In order to be successful when achieving your goals your words and actions must align therefore it is imperative that you choose them wisely.

With respect to reaching long term health and fitness goals you must stop striving to be perfect 100% of the time. The desire for perfection often times leads to disappointment and a feeling of failure. Keep in mind that slow progress is better than no progress; look toward consistency as your goal. That said the weekend shouldn't be used as an excuse to cheat on your food plan and undo all your hard work, nor should you be skipping multiple exercise sessions every week. Remember, if you "kinda, sorta" try, you can expect "kinda, sorta" results.

Realize you must be completely and totally honest with yourself if you are going to move forward and achieve your fitness objectives. Regularly ask yourself if your behavior and your goals are in line. If so keep going, if not modify your actions. You must consistently commit yourself to making choices to live a healthy lifestyle. Consistently eat well, workout, get proper rest and surround yourself with like-minded people. Strive for progress not perfection.

THE KAIZEN PRINCIPLE

The Kaizen Principle is a Japanese concept that was popularized in North America by Dr. W. Edwards Deming. It is based on the premise that results toward any goal come from many small changes accumulated over time. Goals that you once thought were beyond your reach can be attained if practiced gradually, continuously, and constantly.

Take a moment to assess your fitness goals and start to break them down into less significant and seemingly indiscernible pieces. For example, adding exercise such as walking to your daily routine can be addressed by this systematic and persistent approach. The principle of Kaizen will guide you to start slow perhaps walking briskly 10 minutes once a day for a week, then working your way the following week to 12 minutes, then to 14 minutes, and so on.

Be inventive and think outside of the box as you begin to put this concept into action. Keep in mind that you are trying to implement constant and moderate improvement toward your goals. If you want something you've never had, then you've got to do something you've never done. Acknowledge and affirm that the goal is not only achievable, but that failure is impossible.

MEASURING AND ASSESSING YOUR PROGRESS

Changing lifelong, deep-rooted habits will take some time and it can be easy to convince yourself that you are not making positive gains. Therefore, at the onset of your journey you will need to take baseline measurements to track the progress of your efforts.

The intention of these measurements is to be fully aware of the direction you are moving; it's easy to convince yourself that you're not making headway. With regularly scheduled measurements you can assess your transformation and evaluate your course of action. Is what you are doing effective and moving you closer to your goals or do you need to make a few tweaks to perfect and individualize your plan? If the plan isn't working, change the plan not the goal.

Not everyone requires the same frequency; your choice will depend on your objectives. If you have bigger goals, you may want to measure weekly to help keep you in the driver's seat and see where progress is happening or where changes may be in order. If you have more modest goals you may want to check in monthly not relying on the numbers; instead check in with how you feel, how much more energetic you are, and how your clothes fit.

Losing weight does not always advance in a direct and continuous manner. Accomplishments most likely will be followed by plateaus. You may lose steadily for a few weeks, then stagnate, and then move forward again the week after. Not being where you want to be right now has little to do with your future. If you follow a healthy eating and exercise plan, and remain honest with yourself the changes will come and your goals will be realized.

GIRTH MEASUREMENTS

Girth measurements will help you keep track of the changes in your body circumference. With baseline measurements you will be able to quickly and easily scrutinize if you are making strides toward your goals.

At the beginning and throughout your journey to health and wellness regular assessments are important; you will need to measure your body to determine if what you are doing is working for you or if adjustments to your food and exercise plan need to be made. Not everyone will desire the same frequency; some people like to evaluate their progress every 1 to 2 weeks, while others may opt for monthly measurements.

An inexpensive cloth measuring tape is sufficient but you must be sure to measure with consistent tightness for accuracy. For more precise functionality you can purchase a retractable body tape measure; an affordable tool that encircles the body part applying uniform tension for more dependable readings.

Always measure yourself at the same time of the day; I encourage clients to do so first thing in the morning on an empty stomach. Measuring yourself any time other than that can throw things completely off because any amount of eating, drinking, sweating, and bathroom habits over the course of the day will destroy any sense of accuracy.

NECK: measure just below the Adam's apple.

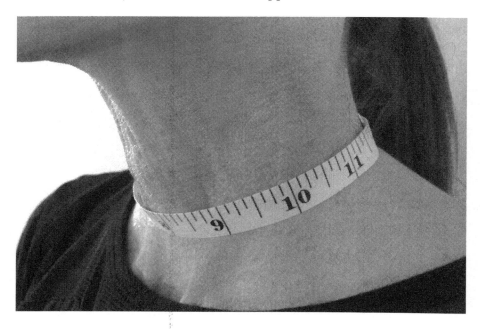

SHOULDER: measure the widest part of the shoulder.

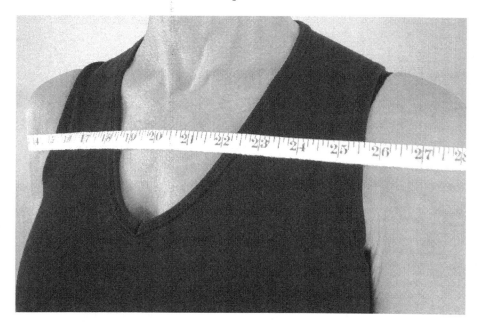

CHEST: measure at the widest point after exhalation.

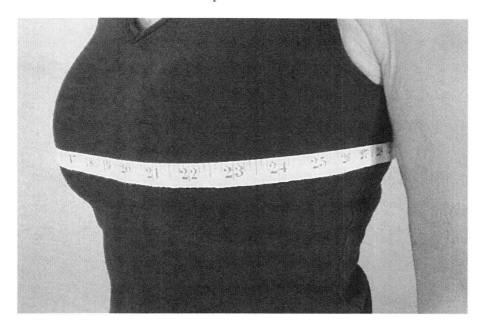

ARM: measure between the elbow and shoulder.

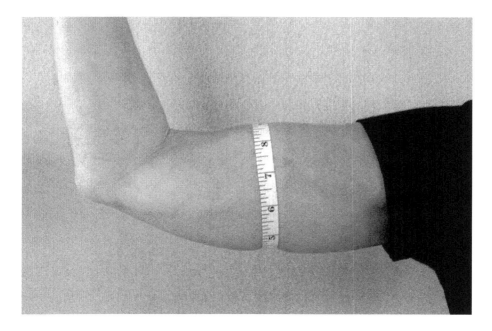

WAIST: measure at the belly button after exhalation.

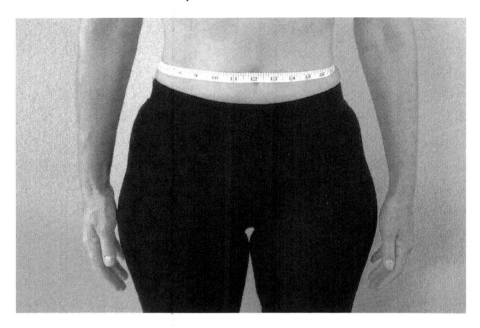

HIP: measure around the widest point of the buttocks.

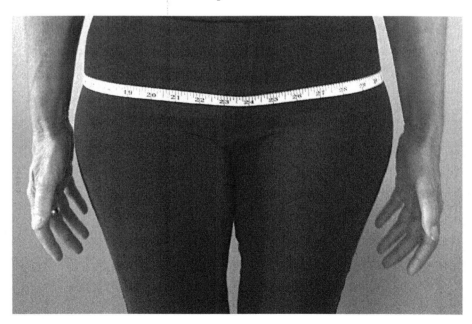

THIGH: measure around the widest point.

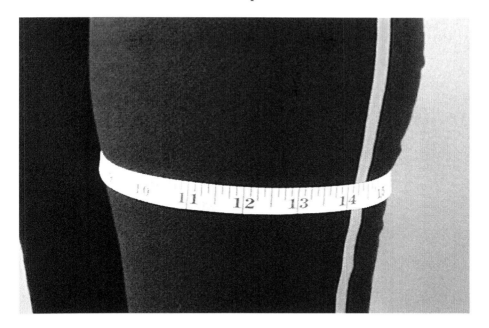

CALF: measure around the widest point.

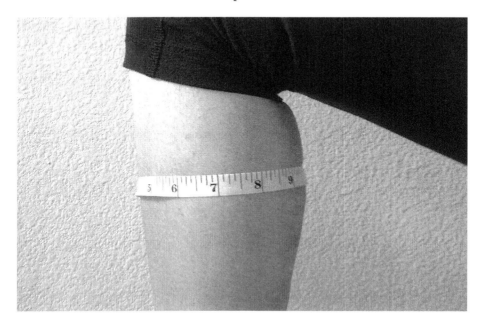

Your Measurements:

Date:

Neck:

Shoulders:

Chest:

Arms   Right: Left:

Waist:

Hips:

Thighs   Right: Left:

Calves   Right: Left:

THE SCALE AND YOU

Measuring your weight is the most common way to assess changes in your body, but bear in mind this isn't just a numbers game. Have you ever heard the claim that a pound of muscle weighs more than a pound of fat? Completely false! A pound is a pound, whether it's sand, feathers, or flour. Muscle has a much greater density than fat; a pound of fat takes up about four times the space of muscle tissue. This explains why it's possible to look and feel slimmer even if your body weight stays the same and the scale doesn't reflect a significant weight loss.

Don't wait until you are a certain weight to be happy. Remember numbers don't tell the whole story. You are modifying long-lived habits to improve your overall health and wellness; the weight will come off naturally with better food choices and increased activity.

You can purchase a simple and accurate digital scale at your local retailer for around $30. Use the scale as one way to begin to track your progress and as a mechanism to keep you honest to you.

As suggested when recording girth measurements weigh yourself at the same time of the day and first thing in the morning on an empty stomach to maintain accuracy. Weighing yourself any time other than that can throw things completely off because of normal bodily functions and routine personal habits.

The frequency at which you weigh yourself is up to you. Some people like to weigh themselves daily. It helps keep them motivated and accountable; they require the daily reminder in order to stay on their plan for healthy eating and incorporating more exercise into their routine. For others a daily weigh-in can be discouraging as it may magnify normal and minor fluctuations caused by water retention or the lack of bowel movement and lead to an unhealthy obsession with the scale.

Only you can decide how often to weigh yourself and what works best for you. Weighing yourself is only one of the many useful tools for tracking your wellness goals. And no matter how good your tools, they aren't what get you the results, following your plan consistently is.

Your Weight:

Date:

Time:

BODY MASS INDEX (BMI)

Research has shown that BMI is highly correlated with the gold-standard approach for measuring body fat. BMI interprets relative height to weight ratio and is a simple way to screen who might be at greater risk of health problems due to their weight.

BMI can be inaccurate for people who are very fit or athletic because their high muscle mass can list them as overweight, even though their body fat percentages are healthy. Taking that into consideration it is an excellent tool for the general population as most people are not athletes, and for most people, BMI is a very good gauge of their level of body fat.

You can determine your BMI by using the index formula:

[Weight in lbs. ÷ (Height in inches x Height in inches)] x 703 = BMI

Example: Weight = 150 lbs., Height = 5'5" (65")

Calculation: [150 ÷ (65 x 65)] x 703 = 24.96

Or quickly and easily determine your BMI by visiting the National Heart Lung and Blood Institute (NHLBI) website for automated calculation:

www.nhlbi.nih.gov/health/educational/lose_wt/BMI/bmicalc.htm

NATIONAL INSTITUTES OF HEALTH BMI STANDARDS

Underweight   Less than 18.5

Normal   18.5 – 24.9

Overweight   25.0 – 29.9

Obese   30.0 or greater

Calculate your BMI:

[Weight in lbs. ÷ (Height in inches x Height in inches)] x 703 = BMI

Where do you fall in the National Standards?

PHOTOGRAPHS

Because some people aren't motivated or satisfied by numbers and they see themselves in the mirror everyday it can be hard to notice the changes as they are happening. It's only when they see themselves 'before' and 'after' that they can see the progress that's occurred. Therefore, while working toward looking and feeling better it's important to document your visual progress. The changes can be so incremental that it's easy to lose sight of the way you appeared at the beginning and how you look throughout your journey.

I strongly encourage you to document the changes by taking photographs of your 'before' physique and monthly thereafter. Take photos from the front and back, as well as left and right side. When you are serious about reaching your goals and are adhering to sound nutritional choices and exercise habits the photos will reveal significant changes and your progress will be obvious.

PREVENTIVE CARE

I am not a doctor, nor do I pretend to be. I steer clear of medical recommendations and will always defer any type of medical questions to the expert, your personal care physician. Before embarking on any wellness plan you should schedule an appointment with your health care provider to discuss what screenings and exams you need. Your age, overall mental and physical condition, family history, lifestyle choices such as what you eat, how active you are, and whether you smoke are some of the factors that will impact your need for healthcare services.

Preventive care is one of the most important steps you can take to manage your health. Regular checkups can help you and your doctor identify lifestyle changes you can make to avoid certain conditions. Developing a strategic plan with clear objectives and following through with the recommended preventive services of your personal care physician are the keys to over-all well-being.

It's time to take charge of your health. By getting the right screenings, services, and treatments, you will be making strides toward living a longer and more vibrant life.

Recognize and know that you are amazing and unique. You have something to offer this world that no one else can. No matter what is happening in your life, whether you are going through good times or times of difficulty, you can accomplish the dreams in your heart. Love yourself and use positive words of encouragement. Compliment strangers and make others smile. Speak from a loving heart and shine with joy.

—Author Unknown

IN HEALTH

- Consider the reason you are eating. Is it an emotional need or physical hunger? If hunger isn't the problem, food will not be the answer. Accept that your journey will require discipline and willpower choosing between what you want now and what you want the most.

- Begin your day with a positive attitude. Wake up in the morning recognizing that you have 24 brand new hours ahead of you and vow to be present and live each moment to the fullest.

- Acknowledge that your choices determine your future; your life can only change by the amount of responsibility you are willing to take for it. If you're searching for that one person that will change your life, take a look in the mirror.

- Positive self-talk is empowering; what you focus on will become your reality. If you realized how powerful your thoughts were you would never think a negative thought again.

- Define your goals and set a date for realization; they should have genuine emotional appeal and be important to you. The only thing standing between you and your goals is the bullshit story you keep telling yourself.

- Shoot for consistency making constant, moderate progress your objective; quit expecting your results to be instant, dramatic, and spectacular! You should be striving for progress not perfection.

- Document your progress with baseline assessments including girth measurements, weight, body mass index, and photographs. Making strides on your journey to wellness can be so incremental that it is easy to lose sight of where you began.

- Take charge of your health by scheduling an appointment with your personal care physician. Together establish a sensible plan based on your current level of fitness and gradually move toward a more energetic and abundant lifestyle.

Download and print your free companion workbook at
www.judymolinaro.com/p/workbook.

Right Food

What you put at the end of your fork is more powerful medicine than anything you will ever find at the bottom of a pill bottle.

Mark Hyman, MD

If you are serious about weight loss and getting fit you need to be completely honest with yourself about how much and what you're really eating each day. No more excuses. If you're not hungry enough to eat an apple, you're not really hungry, you're bored.

If you want to be healthy you need to eat real food. What do I mean by "real food"? Real food doesn't have ingredients; real food is ingredients. If it ever needed sun, dirt, or water it is real food.

Essentially what it boils down to is eat like crap, look and feel like crap. Big food companies and franchises have done a really great job of convincing the American public that they can cook better than we can for ourselves. You cannot eat off the dollar menu and look like a million bucks.

ESSENTIAL NUTRIENTS

There are 6 essential nutrients that are necessary in order to maintain and develop a healthy body: Proteins, Carbohydrates, Fats, Vitamins, Minerals, and Water.

Proteins are essential for growth, the building of new tissue, and the repair of injured or broken-down tissue. Proteins provide amino acids and are derived from both animal and plant foods; lean meats, fish, eggs, dairy, legumes, and protein supplements. While it's easy to grab a protein bar or make a protein shake it's best to get as many whole food meals as possible. No powder, bar, or supplement can come close to matching the vitamins and minerals that are inherent to whole food. Protein provides 4 calories per gram.

Carbohydrates are the body's main source of raw material for energy; they are classified as either simple or complex. Carbohydrates provide 4 calories per gram.

Simple Carbohydrates elevate blood sugar levels rapidly. These "empty calories" are often lacking in vitamins and minerals. Typical examples include sugar, soda, fruit juice, cookies and candy. Avoid when possible.

Complex Carbohydrates contain fiber, which slows digestion and provides many nutrients that your body needs. They can be dense; like bread, pasta, rice, potatoes, corn, legumes, and fruit, or non-dense; like broccoli, spinach, kale, squash, cucumber, lettuce, and tomatoes.

Fats are a necessary part of a balanced diet and are needed for the absorption of fat soluble vitamins (A, D, E, and K) as well as for the synthesis of hormones and cell membranes. They are the most concentrated source of energy in the diet, furnishing 9 calories per gram.

Vitamins are essential for normal metabolism, growth and development, and regulation of cell function. They work together with enzymes and other substances that are necessary for a healthy life.

Minerals are required by the body in small amounts. Your body uses minerals for many different jobs, including building bones, making hormones and regulating your heartbeat.

Water is the most abundant substance in your body and makes up approximately 65 percent of your total bodyweight. Your body uses water in all its cells, organs, and tissues to help regulate its temperature and maintain other bodily functions.

UNDERSTANDING NUTRITION LABELS

Nutrition Facts panels can look promising but they can also come with a lengthy ingredient list. Be skeptical of media hype; Big Food and its marketing machine is not your friend. Many processed foods are opportunistically named "Fit", "Free", "Healthy", "Lean", "Lite", and "Low". Don't fall for deceptive marketing. If they have taken something out you better believe they have put something in to satisfy taste, mouth feel, and shelf life. These additives provide flavor and texture but cheat our senses into believing we are getting better food than we actually are.

Products labeled "made from" or "made with" natural ingredients are often times nothing more than well merchandised junk food. Most processed foods are made from natural ingredients. Even food that is labeled "organic" is not always a healthy choice if it is highly processed; think twice before purchasing "organic junk food".

As well, the US Food and Drug Administration (FDA) allows the nutrition facts on food labels to be inaccurate by up to 20%. Your diet should be mostly high quality, minimally processed, whole food sources.

Serving Size - Many food labels serving sizes are ridiculously small, unrealistic, and not the amount of food a person would customarily consume in a typical sitting. That's because they are based on outdated information going back as far as the 70's when people ate a lot less and the calculated manipulation of the facts.

For example, a leading brand of coffee creamer suggests that a serving size is 1 tablespoon. It is hard to believe that this small amount of product would be considered a serving as many people typically use several times that amount. As well, many people mistakenly assume that small packages are a single serving when in fact the manufacturer may suggest they be several servings.

Calories - Think of calories as the energy food delivers to your body. This energy is what your body burns through physical activity. When you burn the same amount of energy as you consume, you maintain your weight. If you consume more energy than you burn, you're going to gain weight. And if you consume less energy than you burn, you're going to lose weight.

Eating nutritious foods is imperative for health but you must pay overall attention to the amount you are taking in. For example, the average person cannot eat an unlimited amount of lean meat, whole grains, fruits and vegetables in one day even if what they are eating is deemed healthy and expect to maintain or lose weight.

With distorted serving sizes and oversized portions calories can add up very quickly. If you take in more calories than you expend, you will store the excess as fat.

Fat - As we discussed earlier fat is an essential part of a balanced diet. The only fat that should be off limits is trans-fat. Based on scientific review of partially hydrogenated oils (PHO's) the US Food and Drug Administration (FDA) indicates they are not generally recognized as safe for human consumption. The good news is that the FDA has announced its decision to ban PHO's and manufacturers have until June 18, 2018 to adjust their products.

Trans-fats are an artificially produced fat used to extend the shelf life of products like baked goods, margarine, cake mixes, frozen dinners, etc. and guess what…coffee creamer! At first glance many processed foods appear to be trans-fat free. However, it can be very deceiving; the FDA only requires food manufacturers to list the amount of trans-fat in the product if it is higher than a half a gram per serving. Remember that the serving size is being determined by the manufacturer and in many cases it is ridiculously small often to manipulate facts and dupe the consumer.

Be aware when reading labels, you are dealing with a "food marketing machine". Even if it claims to be trans-fat free, it could still have a high amount of trans-fat in a typical and customary serving. You must take the time to read the ingredients label and look for partially hydrogenated oils.

Saturated Fat is found mainly in animal foods like meat, and dairy products. It can also be found in tropical oils derived from plants; look for palm oil, palm kernel oil, and coconut oil.

Polyunsaturated Fat and Monounsaturated Fat is found in fish, soybeans, avocados, liquid vegetable oils, nuts and seeds.

Cholesterol - The Dietary Guidelines Advisory Committee (DGAC) has concluded cholesterol is not a nutrient of concern. Available evidence shows no considerable relationship between dietary intake of cholesterol and blood cholesterol.

The theory has had remarkable staying power despite years of doubts from prominent scientists. The narrow-minded focus on fat has distorted our diet and contributed to the biggest health crisis facing America today. For an in depth look at the history of this long maligned nutrient see Time Magazine's June 23, 2014 report "Don't Blame Fat".

Sodium - The Dietary Guidelines Advisory Committee (DGAC) recommend an upper limit for sodium consumption of less than 2,400 milligrams per day which equals approximately 1 teaspoon for adults. The average person gets 12% of their daily intake of salt from whole food (meat, vegetables, and fruit), 11% from the salt shaker, and 77% from processed foods.

A best-selling canned soup that may be in your pantry packs a wallop at 2,225 mg of sodium per can. The manufacturer of this product claims that there are 2.5 servings per can; a much smaller serving size than would typically be eaten at one sitting. You must be diligent and pay close attention to labels if and when you are consuming processed foods.

If you eat cured meats, you've probably encountered sodium nitrate or sodium nitrite. Both chemicals act as food preservatives and add a red or pink color to processed meats. Most of these meats are high in sodium and can disrupt a healthy diet; it's best to limit the amount you consume.

Total Carbohydrate on the label includes all types of carbohydrates; fiber, sugar, and complex carbohydrates. Beneath the Total Carbohydrate line there will be two or three sub categories-fiber (both soluble and insoluble may be listed), sugars, and sugar alcohols if it is present. You may notice that these figures do not add up to the total. This is because complex carbohydrates are not typically listed on food labels. Therefore, any missing carbohydrates can be complex; that is the ones naturally present in the food as well as the non-digestible additives, such as stabilizers and thickening agents so prevalent in processed foods.

Any flour without "whole grain" in front of it has been refined. Whole grain means that all three parts of the grain kernel (or seed) are used; including the nutritious bran, endosperm, and germ. Whole grains are a nutritional powerhouse; higher in vitamins, minerals and fiber than refined grains, which are processed to remove all but the starchy endosperm. Whole wheat flours or foods made with whole wheat flour, such as breads and rolls, are not whole grain products because of the way they are produced. Don't be fooled by imaginatively labeled products. Whole wheat, organic flour, multigrain, stoneground, durum wheat etc. are not as nutritious as foods labeled as being whole grain.

You may also see terms such as "net carbohydrates" or "impact carbohydrates" on processed food labels. These terms have no legal definition from the FDA and are used as a marketing tool to sell products.

Dietary Fiber, also known as roughage, is a complex carbohydrate found in plant foods, such as whole grains, fruits, vegetables, legumes and nuts. It is the indigestible part of the plant foods that pushes through our digestive system, absorbing water along the way and helps maintain bowel regularity. Fiber is the only type of carbohydrate that your body cannot digest, so it does not provide energy or increase blood sugar levels.

Soluble Fiber dissolves in water. It changes as it goes through the digestive tract, where it is fermented by bacteria. As it absorbs water it becomes gelatinous slowing digestion.

Insoluble Fiber does not dissolve in water. As it goes through the digestive tract it does not change its form. It adds bulk to the stool and helps food pass more quickly through the stomach and intestines.

Sugars - Several types of sugar exist, such as sucrose, fructose and lactose, which are the scientific names for table, fruit, and milk sugar, respectively. Take note that grams of sugar on the label does not distinguish between added and natural sugars. For instance, a banana has no added sugar but contains sugar naturally. In order to determine how much sugar is in each serving divide the number of sugar grams by 4 to get the number of teaspoons per serving.

Now is the time to go to your refrigerator and look at a few items you may have in stock and see how many teaspoons of sugar you are eating per serving. For example, while consumers tend to think of juice as a healthy drink it's really refined fruit with the water and fiber removed. When the water is removed to make it taste better it becomes a denser source of sugar.

High-fructose corn syrup (HFCS) is a manmade sweetener that has gotten a lot of press in recent years. It is found in a wide range of processed foods, from ketchup and cereals to crackers and salad dressings. It also sweetens just about all of the regular soda Americans drink. Products with HFCS are sweeter and cheaper than products made with cane sugar. This allowed for the average soda size to balloon from eight ounces to 20 ounces with little financial costs to manufacturers but great human costs of increased obesity, diabetes and chronic disease.

More and more packaged foods are sweetened with a baffling array of sugars. Among them are beet sugar, cane juice, corn sweetener, dextrose, fructose, lactose, glucose, maltose, barley malt, malt extract, and rice syrup. The takeaway is to be diligent and read labels. If you want to have some sugar, that's fine, have a little sugar, but control the portion size by adding it to your food yourself.

Artificial sweeteners, such as Sucralose (Splenda), Saccharin (Sweet 'N Low), Aspartame (NutraSweet, Equal, AminoSweet), and Acesulfame K (Sunnet) can cut down on calories in foods like yogurt and beverages. But studies warn that some artificial sweeteners can be dangerous in large quantities; it's best to consume artificial sweeteners in moderation.

Sugar Alcohols come from plant products such as fruits and berries. If a manufacturer uses the term "sugar free" or "no added sugar," they must list the grams of sugar alcohols. They are found most commonly in hard candies, cookies, chewing gums, and soda. As well they are frequently used in toothpaste, mouthwash, and throat lozenges.

The sugar alcohols commonly found in foods are sorbitol, mannitol, xylitol, isomalt, and hydrogenated starch hydrolysates. These ingredients were given this consumer-friendly name because part of their structure resembles sugar and part is similar to alcohol. These sugar substitutes provide somewhat fewer calories, 0 to 3 calories per gram compared to 4 calories per gram for table sugar (sucrose). They are not always well absorbed and may cause bloating, diarrhea, and even have a laxative effect.

Protein is a necessary nutrient. All foods made from meat, poultry, seafood, beans and peas, eggs, processed soy products, nuts, and seeds are considered part of the protein foods group.

Be mindful that many processed forms of protein that we may initially identify as whole foods can contain additives, preservatives, and carbohydrates. Take the time to read the ingredients label on products you are considering purchasing. Common examples are egg substitutes, imitation crab, and frozen meats and fish.

Most adults don't have any problem getting enough protein in their daily diet. However, if getting all of your protein from whole food sources is not practical you may want to occasionally substitute protein powders. Protein powders come in many forms; whey, casein, soy, pea, rice and hemp are most common. Keep in mind these supplements are highly processed and their intake should be limited.

Percent Daily Value recommended intakes of nutrients vary by age and gender. These daily values were developed by the FDA to help consumers determine the level of various nutrients in a standard serving of food in relation to their approximate requirement for it. The label actually provides the %DV so that you can see what percentage a serving of the product contributes to reaching the daily value.

To get the most benefit from Percent Daily Values don't get caught up in the numbers; use them to choose foods high in vitamins, minerals and fiber and to limit foods high in fat and sodium.

Ingredients lists are a good way to know exactly what packaged food contains and is a useful tool for the consumer. The ingredient list matters most because you can technically create a food product that "hits all the right numbers" using highly processed, minimally nutritious ingredients. Ingredients are listed in descending order by weight, meaning the first ingredient makes up the largest proportion of the food.

Check the ingredients list to spot things you want to avoid like trans-fats, artificial sugars, refined flours, and preservatives. You may be surprised by what you find added to what you assumed to be "whole" food. For instance, many popular dried fruits have been processed with oil and sugar.

Be conscientious when shopping; don't fall for the manufacturer's clever marketing gimmicks. Always use a discerning eye when choosing what goes into your grocery cart, your body will thank you.

KITCHEN MAKEOVER

If food is within your reach you will eventually eat it. Rid your home, office, car, or wherever it is that you may keep a stash of unhealthy food choices. You don't have to throw it away, donate it to a food bank, a shelter, or a local church.

Some people would argue that you need to develop willpower and I agree that you do; having personal control is critical. But while you're in the process of learning and developing a sound nutritional lifestyle you do not need to be faced with additional temptations. Why would you want to make the transition any more difficult? Why put yourself in a position to eat heavily processed foods and make regrettable food choices? Why test your willpower?

Most people have enough food stored up to survive an apocalypse. The average pantry in today's home resembles that of a food bunker. How and why did a small storage cabinet in the kitchen turn into a walk-in closet to be envied? It is not uncommon to see large stand-alone refrigerators and freezers in modern kitchens. Where did we ever come up with the idea that we need to buy and store so much processed food?

Shelves are overflowing with bags of cookies, crackers, and chips. They are lined with rows of boxes touting "instant" this and "ready" that; jars of "recipe secrets" and "simple starts"; cans of "heat and serve" and "ultra-convenient ". Freezers filled with "entrée kits", "diet TV dinners", "chicken nuggets", "fish sticks", and "organic junk food". Refrigerators loaded with sugary drinks and fruit juices, dips, dressings, and sauces laden with sugar, sodium, and fat.

It's time to ditch processed food in a dramatic blaze of glory. Your goal is to keep only items that are as close to the original, whole food as possible. Don't try to convince yourself that you can keep bad food within reach and change your habits; breaking bad habits isn't always that easy.

While it's easy to throw out the obviously terrible items like, candy, chips, cookies, soda, and sugar-laden fruit juice it may be more difficult to toss out the frozen pizzas and microwave burritos. You will be more likely to stick with great food choices if you don't have your old staples to fall back on. Don't expect to see a change unless you make one.

Evaluate and consider the foods you used to think of as okay with new eyes, odds are you will be surprised. Read the label and ingredients list and decide to keep the product or toss it out based on its nutritional merit.

It's time to do the dirty work; clean out your pantry, refrigerator, and freezer. You must look at nutrition labels and start to examine and scrutinize each one. Armed with knowledge and a discriminating eye put what you've learned into use.

On a sheet of paper write down the name of the product and answer:

1. What most concerns you about consuming this product?

2. What product can you substitute it with that will be a healthier choice?

GROCERY SHOPPING

Good nutrition starts with smart choices at the grocery store. If you buy good food, you'll eat good food; the key to your success will be a properly stocked pantry. If your life is jam packed with responsibilities having a well-stocked pantry is your best defense; it means you will always have healthy choices available.

Planning your meals ahead of time will help you be efficient when you tackle grocery shopping and you'll be less tempted to buy unhealthy and unnecessary items. Remember to include everything you will need for breakfast, lunch, dinner, and snacks.

A lot of people say it costs too much to eat healthy, I disagree. The average American family spends nearly as much money on fast food as they do the groceries. With 2/3 of Americans overweight it's clear our portion sizes and food choices have gotten out of control. You won't be eating out, you'll be eating less, and you won't be buying junk food so your grocery dollars will go further than ever before.

Environmental psychologist, Paco Underhill the author of the book *Why We Buy: The Science of Shopping* reports that two thirds of what we buy in the supermarket we had no intention of buying. Make your grocery list and stick to it.

Don't shop hungry or you will come home the proud owner of aisle 4! An empty belly often results in impulse purchases that may not be the healthiest.

Try to shop without the distractions of children. Food manufacturers don't blink an eye targeting your children by strategically placing "kid-friendly" processed junk at their eye level with popular cartoon characters on the packaging.

Allow yourself some extra time to read labels; you have the power to determine what goes into your shopping cart, in your home, and in your body. When in doubt, leave it out.

You have probably heard that you should shop the outer perimeter of the store. Every aspect of a stores layout is designed to stimulate shopping so you're not safe using that as your guide. The food industry spends millions of dollars on research to learn how to manipulate us to buy their products. Displays at the end of aisles, treats in the check-out lanes and flashy signs revealing sale items are there to lure you into purchasing products they want you to buy. Deli's overflowing with fried chicken and tubs of potato & macaroni salad, bakeries loaded with sugar and fat laden sweets, cases full of sandwich meats, processed fish & meat, organic junk food, breakfast items, snack cakes, and soda are often found on the outer perimeter.

There are good choices buried in the aisles but don't be an "aisle browser". Make trips down the aisles when you need specific items like tuna, whole grains, nuts, frozen fruits and vegetables.

Use your common sense and new found knowledge; seek out healthy foods, read nutrition labels and don't buy into slick advertising gimmicks. You'll know you're "earthy crunchy" when you don't bother clipping coupons because all the coupons are for food that isn't real.

In order to make shopping faster and easier personalize your grocery list. These will be the things that you buy most often and don't want to forget to have on hand and available for meals and snacks. Keeping a checklist of the items that you want to stock your pantry and refrigerator with will make grocery shopping effortless.

You can easily create this list on your computer; print out several copies and each time you need a new shopping list you have one at your fingertips. Simply add things to it that are on sale or are special purchases for preparing a particular recipe or for just trying something new.

FOOD PREPARATION

Lose weight in the kitchen, get fit in the gym. I cannot emphasize this point enough. You must eat your own home cooked food as often as you can. Stopping to grab food on the go, heading out to lunch with co-workers, nibbling from the goodies left in the lunchroom and too many dinners out will derail your efforts. Don't spend your day in a food coma. When making choices ask yourself "Is what I'm about to do going to get me closer to or further away from my goal?"

If you are like most people you have a job, commitments, responsibilities, and distractions that will take you off course every day. You've heard it before, if you fail to plan, your plan will fail. When you have the beginnings of healthy meals started, you are much less likely to reach for junk food or swing into the drive through. If you get the messy, time consuming work of food preparation out of the way you will always have access to fresh, nutritious meals quickly and easily.

There is no right or wrong way to prepare food ahead of time; don't get bogged down into thinking it has to be done a certain way. When starting out, don't try and prepare your entire weekly menu plan ahead of time as this may overwhelm you. Look at your meal plan for the next few days and work from there. The first few weeks try preparing a couple of meals ahead of time and as you get comfortable with the process you can do more.

Involve the family, pass on the knowledge so they will make healthy choices and learn to practice good dietary habits. I find that spending a couple of hours at a time in the kitchen preparing a few days of meals ahead is a huge time saver during the week. There are some things you will always want to have ready to eat. I fill my refrigerator with things like hard-boiled eggs, whole grain pasta and brown rice, steamed and roasted vegetables, chopped fruits and salads, and soups and stews. Remember good nutritional choices will be easier to make when meals are readily available.

Having the proper containers, utensils, cooler, and icepacks is a must when preparing food for storage and for meals and snacks to package on the go. I know it sounds ridiculous that I am telling you to buy things like Ziploc bags and food storage containers but not having these simple items handy gives you a perfect excuse for not doing the preparation needed to accomplish your goals. Take inventory of your cabinets and write down what you need to buy in order to organize your efforts.

When can you find the time for meal preparation?

What are some things you can do to streamline the process?

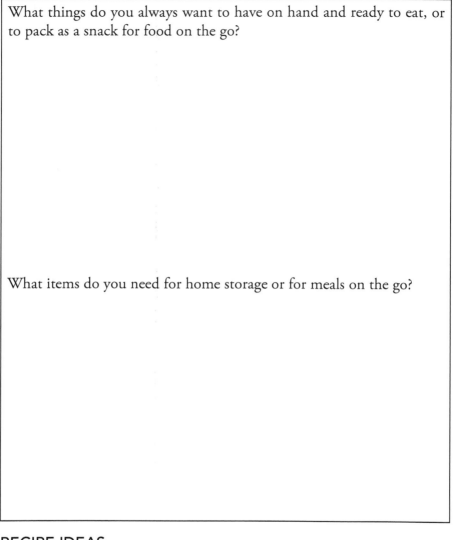

What things do you always want to have on hand and ready to eat, or to pack as a snack for food on the go?

What items do you need for home storage or for meals on the go?

RECIPE IDEAS

A healthy lifestyle involves many choices and you may be feeling a little overwhelmed at this point; please don't let this slow you down. Your success is nothing more than committing to a few simple disciplines practiced every day.

Recipe choices will have a major impact on your health, wellness, and success. Get inspiration for new wholesome foods by searching the internet; it is chock-full of delicious meal ideas. You have a computer, you know how to use it and now you have an understanding of what real food is. Start Googling!

The important thing is to keep it simple. Recipes that require too many odd ingredients and too much preparation time will cause you to lose steam. Narrow down what you are looking for and search for specific meal ideas like grilled meats, crock pot entrees, pressure cooker dishes, roasted vegetables etc. and you will be well on your way to a healthy new you.

Do you have to give up your favorite comfort foods? No, you just need to find ways to fit them into your lifestyle that still helps you lose weight or maintain a healthy weight. You can still enjoy your family favorites by eating them less often, in smaller portions, and served alongside nutritious, whole food choices. As well, look for healthier and more nutritionally sound versions of your family's favorite recipes and include them in your eating plan. Healthy eating is all about balance.

While preparing meals it's important to be conscious of mindless eating; nibbling away hundreds of calories at time, a lick here and a taste there. The combination of I'm hungry, it tastes good, and I'm stressed adds up and by the time you are ready to sit down for dinner you're already full. It's hard to keep track of what you've eaten when you swipe bites and it's easy to shrug them off as nothing resulting in "food amnesia". At the end of the day these excess calories will pack on the pounds; the logical conclusion is to not eat while cooking.

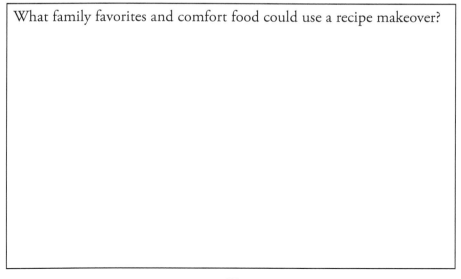

What family favorites and comfort food could use a recipe makeover?

PORTION CONTROL

Americans spend more than $60 billion every year trying to lose weight. The diet industries advice and products offer virtually no long-term return on investment. Most people who participate in weight-loss programs regain about one-third of the weight lost during the next year and are typically back to baseline weight in three to five years. Diets are a fast way to make temporary progress and calorie counting is tedious and unsustainable.

Portion control is the key to keeping calories in check and is the foundation for successful weight loss and weight management. Many of us don't understand what a healthy portion size is, and for good reason. Research reveals the history of food portions have been on the rise since the 20th century and found that portions are much bigger than they were in the past, up to 2-5 times bigger, to be exact.

For most people portion size is anything but obvious. When most people sit down to eat they tend to underestimate how much they are actually eating. The good news is that with a little practice, portion control is easy to understand and carry out; it will help you achieve your goals and establish healthy habits for a lifetime of success.

The first step to portion control is learning the correct serving size. Your hand corresponds closely to your body size making it a convenient and distinctive way to measure food consumption.

PERSONALIZE YOUR PORTIONS

Protein Portion

Your open palm determines your protein portion. This palm sized portion should be equivalent to the diameter and thickness of your hand.

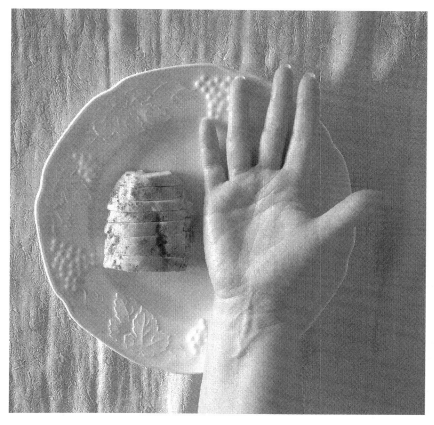

Amount   Women: 1 palm size serving with each meal
Men: 2 palm size servings with each meal

Examples   Chicken, turkey, beef
Salmon, tuna, cod
Greek yogurt, cottage cheese, eggs
Tofu

Vegetable Portion: Non-Dense

Your closed fist represents your non-dense vegetable portion.

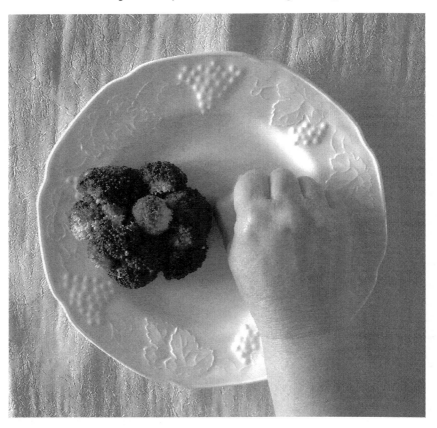

Amount   Women: 1 fistful with each meal
           Men: 2 fistfuls with each meal

Examples   Broccoli, kale, lettuce, asparagus, peppers,
           yellow squash, tomatoes, spinach

Carbohydrate Portion: Dense

Your cupped hand determines your dense carbohydrate portion.

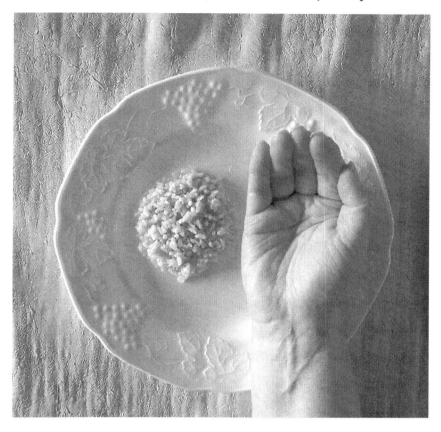

Amount	Women: 1 cupped handful with each meal
	Men: 2 cupped handfuls with each meal

Examples	Bread, cereal, pasta, rice, oats, potatoes, corn, beans, fruit

Fat Portion

Your thumb determines your fat portion.

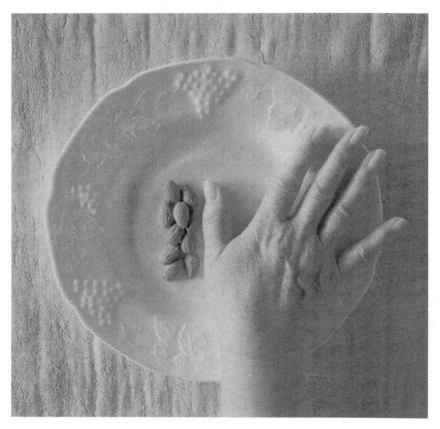

Amount   Women: 1 thumb sized serving with each meal
         Men: 2 thumb sized servings with each meal

Examples   Nuts and nut butters, seeds, olives, butter, oils

Keep in mind this model serves as a starting point. Stay flexible and adjust your portions based on your level of activity. Take into account what you have just done or how active you are going to be in the next few hours. Be honest with yourself; don't use your answer as a convenient excuse to overeat.

While it is essential that you consume enough protein to support growth and recovery, carbohydrates (dense and non-dense) to deliver energy to your body, and fats for many basic body functions you cannot lose weight efficiently unless you are in a negative calorie balance. You must be mindful of how much food you are serving yourself; portion control will be the key factor in reaching your healthy weight objectives.

PLATE SIZE

An empty stomach is approximately the size of your fist and can expand up to 10 times its original size. Once expanded, over time, it's less likely to shrink back to its original size. That's why smaller meals and smaller portions are a sensible route to take. Consider the size of your plates and bowls to help you limit your food intake at each meal.

Most of us eat with our eyes and if given a large plate or bowl will be tempted to fill it and compelled to eat it. It's time to resign from the clean plate club.

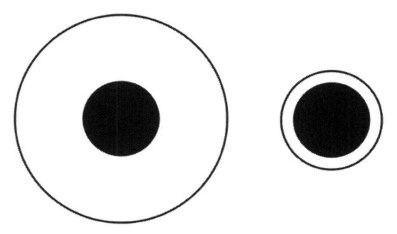

The solid black circles above are exactly the same size. The illusion created is that the solid circle on the right is bigger.

In the 1960's, dinner plates were roughly 9 inches in diameter; in the 1980's they grew to around 10 inches, by the year 2000, the average dinner plate was 11 inches in diameter, and now, it's not unusual to find dishes that are 12 inches or larger.

If you choose smaller plates and bowls you are likely to be satisfied with the portion served and be able to put the fork down when you are 80% full, not when you are stuffed or the plate is empty.

Start paying attention to your appetite and fullness cues, cultivate an intuitive eating style. Many of us eat far too quickly and want to eat to the point of being full. Take your time and experience the action of eating; slow down, turn off the TV, push away from the computer, and eliminate distractions.

It takes roughly 20 minutes for our satiety mechanisms to kick in. The communication from our stomach to our brain is slow and because of this if you eat too quickly you're likely to eat too much. Give your brain time to register that you are content and can stop eating now.

MEALS AND SNACKS

Try to eat four to five times a day; two to three meals is not enough if you are following this portion control model. Active people tend to get hungry every three to four hours. Two of these meals should be considered as snacks to get you through to your next meal and to prevent you from getting too hungry which can make you susceptible to overeating.

Don't fall prey to portion distortion! A snack is a mini-meal, not a meal; your portion sizes need to be kept to a minimum. A hard-boiled egg and a thumb of almonds, a fistful of raw vegetables and a thumb of hummus, a cupped hand of sliced apples and a thumb of peanut butter, or a palm of yogurt and cupped hand of berries are all healthy and nutritious snack ideas that are great eaten anytime of the day.

When it comes to snacks, plan ahead to ensure you have healthy foods available when you need them. Choosing foods from different groups will help balance your diet and go a long way toward providing the nutrients you need for good health and top performance.

Eating small, frequent meals can fuel your body for quality workouts and good health; blood sugar and insulin levels will be controlled and thus your energy level. By supplying your body with a consistent and frequent amount of just the right number of calories, its need to store fat is lessened. Comparatively, when you eat infrequently your body identifies a famine situation and the food you eat is stored as body fat in preparation for the famine to come by lowering your metabolism.

Your metabolism is the chemical process that occurs within your body in order to maintain life and includes all the things your body does to turn food into energy and keep you going; it can be high, low, or somewhere in the middle.

> Make a list of convenient and healthy snack ideas that you enjoy; always have them on hand to satisfy your hunger and nutritional needs.

WATER

Water is your body's principal chemical component. It makes up approximately 65% of your weight and is involved in every type of cellular process in your body. When you're dehydrated, they all run less efficiently and that includes your metabolism.

Think of it like your car; if you have oil, water, and gas, it will run more smoothly. It's the same with your body. It can be difficult for the body to tell the difference between hunger and thirst. So if you're feeling an acute sense of hunger, you might just be dehydrated.

Every day you lose water through your breath, perspiration, urine and bowel movements. How do you know if you're getting enough water to keep your metabolism performing at peak efficiency? The formula used to be one size fits all, eight, 8-ounce glasses of water a day. Experts agree that has changed; they now believe it depends on your size, weight, activity level, and the climate where you live.

Generally speaking, every day you should drink between half an ounce to an ounce of water for each pound you weigh. For example, if you weigh 160 pounds, that would be 80 to 160 ounces of water a day. If you're living in a hot climate and exercising a lot, you will be on the higher end of that range; if you're in a cooler climate and mostly sedentary, you will need less.

While the water you drink should make the main contribution to your daily requirements, foods that contain water may also play a role. Approximately 80% of our water intake comes from drinking, and the other 20% comes from food. While 20% may seem like a lot of fluid, many common food items are mostly water. For example, a banana is about 74% water, while a pear is 84% and watermelon is 92%. The water content of many vegetables including lettuce, spinach, tomatoes, and zucchini is more than 90%. Even meat, poultry and fish contribute to fluid intake. For example, flounder is 79% water, chicken 69%, extra-lean ground beef 63%, and eggs 75%.

Although difficult, it is possible to drink too much water; water toxicity is a real threat. During exercise that results in a large amount of sweat loss drinking too much water could lead to mineral imbalances and even death. This is why sports drinks containing carbohydrates, proteins and minerals are consumed during long-duration exercise like marathons. However, for most activities drinking regular water throughout the day is enough to meet your hydration needs.

Calculate your daily minimum and maximum water needs:

One half ounce to one ounce of water for each pound you weigh.

JOURNALING

What if I told you that by making one simple addition to your daily routine, you could double your weight loss? While it may sound too good to be true, studies have shown that people who keep food journals are more successful at losing weight and keeping it off. The American Journal of Preventive Medicine reports that people keeping a food diary six days a week lost about twice as much weight as those who kept records one day a week or less.

How is it that the simple act of keeping a food diary will become one of your most powerful weight-management tools? Writing down and keeping track of your food intake increases your awareness of when, what, and how much you are eating. It holds you accountable and helps you cut down on mindless munching; many of us want food to not count because we're just finishing off the broken cookies in the bag, or nibbling while preparing dinner.

The lack of adherence is the number one reason people fail when trying to lose or maintain weight. For some people the simple act of having to record every bite helps discourage overeating because they don't want to have to write it in their journal. Additionally, food diaries help identify areas where changes need to be made by unveiling patterns and triggers to avoid, such as not eating enough throughout the day and then overeating at night, or overeating when drinking alcohol.

Choose a method of journaling that fits into your life. It might be a simple spiral bound notebook, an online program, or an app on your Smartphone. The point is to keep it handy; filling it out every day, and logging your food intake right away so that you are accurate. The basic elements should include the date, time, what you ate, and the portion size.

It's important to record everything even if it seems painful. It can be tempting to avoid recording an unplanned indulgence, excessive nibbling, or a binge episode. Write down things you think may have influenced your food choice such as how you felt physically, emotionally, if you were rushed for time, or if you had a suitable meal readily available.

Additionally, be sure to include how much water you drank as well as the amount and type of activity and exercise you performed that day.

Record your weight and measurements in your journal at least once a week, preferably the same day and time to track your progress. Remember, you can fundamentally change your body without losing or gaining a pound. This will happen when you lose fat while gaining lean muscle mass when you begin to increase your level of exercise.

Where are you making strides?

Where is there room for improvement?

What could you have done to make better choices?

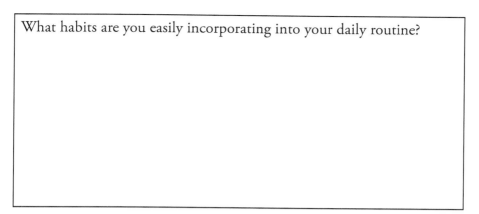

What habits are you easily incorporating into your daily routine?

Your journal will be a useful tool to review; the simple act of acknowledgment and reflection is an important component to your success in reaching your health goals.

EATING AS A FAMILY

Research reveals that not eating together as a family has quantifiable negative effects physically and psychologically.

Sadly, the average American eats one in five meals in their car, one in four Americans eats at least one fast food meal every single day, and the majority of American families report eating a single meal together less than five days a week.

Children who do not eat dinner with their parents at least twice a week are 40% more likely to be overweight compared to those who do. Recent studies indicate that children who eat dinner with their parents five or more days a week eat healthier, have higher grade-point averages and self-esteem, and report being closer with their parents. The studies also link regular family dinners with lowering the rates of high risk teenage behaviors parents fear; smoking, binge drinking, drug use, violence, depression, school problems, eating disorders and sexual activity.

Mealtime is the most predictable way for families to connect and communicate with each other. A recent survey reveals that when asked, American teens were most likely to talk with their parents at dinner. So it's no surprise to learn that when teenagers are asked about the importance of family dinners, they rate them very high on their list of priorities. You should assume that your kids want to have dinner with you.

Feeding your family nutritious food not only makes your children healthier as they grow but will be the foundation for healthy eating patterns once they are living on their own.

Most children like to be involved in family activities and should be encouraged to do so. Many teens view cooking as a way of expressing themselves and may enjoy making a meal or a portion of it. Even young children can participate in meal preparation by sprinkling in a seasoning, stirring a soup, or washing vegetables.

Along with the appreciation for wholesome food and the work that goes into cooking a meal, there are also many social elements that come into play when sharing food as a family. The table can be a welcome environment where children learn how to conduct conversations, observe proper manners, practice social skills, and learn about family culture. Family meals are for nourishment, enjoyment and support; food is best shared and eaten with the people we love!

People are fed by the food industry, which pays no attention to health and treated by people in the health industry, which pays no attention to food.

—Author Unknown

IN HEALTH

- Maintain your health by learning the sources of the 6 essential nutrients. Each and every cell in your body is derived from the food you eat. If you consume junk food, expect a junk body.

- Nutrition labels provide an abundance of data. Food isn't simply calories; it is information; it talks to your DNA. Every time you eat or drink you are either feeding disease or fighting it.

- The kitchen makeover may very well be one of the most difficult tasks you complete. Stop focusing on what you have to give up and focus on what you have to gain! If you don't take care of your body where are you going to live?

- Grocery shopping is the foundation of a healthy diet and will be your catalyst for change. While it may seem daunting at first don't give up, the beginning is always the hardest part. And please don't try to convince me that it costs too much to eat healthy. Millions of people will spend $5 on a fancy coffee but refuse to spend $5 on fruit.

- Food preparation and recipe choices are key to maintaining momentum. You must find time to have nutritious and delicious food ready to grab and go. If not, you are going to be upset by the results you didn't get from the work you didn't do.

- Be mindful of your portion sizes and the dinnerware you are using to serve yourself. Remember, a meal is a meal and a snack is a snack!

- Water is high octane fuel for the body. Be sure to calculate your needs and drink enough to meet your minimum requirements.

- Keeping a journal need not be a chore. Pick a method and do it!

- Celebrate being a family every day. Spend time with your children around the kitchen table to connect and share thoughts.

Download and print your free companion workbook at www.judymolinaro.com/p/workbook.

Right Exercise

Exercise would be so much more rewarding if calories screamed as you burned them!

Author Unknown

In order to lose body fat, look better, and feel energized, you must get moving! Whether you want to lose 15lbs or 50lbs exercise is essential and plays a significant role in your success. You are not going to get the butt you want by sitting on it. If you want more, you've got to be willing to do more and the hardest thing about exercise is to start doing it.

Getting fit is a slow and steady process; being fit is not a destination, it's a way of life. Adhering to regularly scheduled workouts will take commitment, determination and discipline; doing what needs to be done, when it needs to be done, when you don't want to do it. The bottom line is you can't wish for a strong, healthy body, you've got to work for it.

You're probably saying to yourself, "I'll never look like the girl in the magazine." I have news for you; the girl in the magazine doesn't look like the girl in the magazine! You have always been beautiful, decide now to be healthier, fitter and stronger; define success on your own terms.

Your desire will be created when something happens in your life that suddenly changes the way you see yourself in relationship to your future. At any given moment you have the power to change your life and say, "This is not how my story is going to end".

EXCUSES, EXCUSES!

I have never known anyone who after a workout said "I wish I hadn't done that". Or after they began to get stronger, more toned, and realized weight loss said "Boy that was a waste of time". The sooner you shift into action the sooner you will see and feel the results of recurrent exercise. Stop hiding from exercise. Get out of the fitness protection program!

I have been in and out of gyms for nearly 40 years and I think it's safe to say that I have heard just about every excuse there is not to exercise. If you lose the excuses I promise you that you will find the results. The more often you say you can't do something the more reasons you will give yourself to not do it. You don't need outside detractors and cynics; you're killing your dreams all by yourself. Stop being your own worst enemy and start being your own best friend. Don't let someday turn into never.

It's curious that we are willing to make time for something if we are truly motivated. Take a look at yourself; do you make excuses that you are too squeezed for time to make it to the gym or to go for a walk? But easily find time to endlessly surf the internet, go to the movies or happy hour with friends. It's not about having the time; it's about making the time.

There are 168 hours in a week.

   40 hours at work
   56 hours of sleep
   72 hours are leftover

Are you serious? You can't find time to exercise?

I know right now you are coming up with all kinds of reasons why you can't find time to exercise. What are they? Get up off of your butt, get a pen, and write them down right this minute!

It's right about now I know that you are saying "Yeah but you don't understand Judy...blah, blah, blah..." Yes, I do understand! I can think of all kinds of excuses not to work out too, but I do it anyway. If it's important you will find the time, if not you will find an excuse. I can assure you, people much busier than you are working out right now. What are you waiting for?

EXERCISE - WHAT KIND AND HOW MUCH?

I'm often asked "What kind of exercise is the best"? My answer is always the same "Whatever you will commit to and do consistently". The key to successfully incorporating exercise into your already busy and demanding schedule and have it become a routine is to create a program around activities that you enjoy at a time of day that works for you.

Many of us are creatures of habit. We tend to go to the same class at the gym, log onto the same program on the treadmill, and repeatedly practice the same weight lifting exercises and stretches. While regular exercise is good for you, it's important to change up your routine. There are three modalities that you will want to consider alternating between in your workouts; cardiovascular/aerobic exercise, weight training/strength building routines, and flexibility/balance training.

When you include different types of activity both your body and brain reap the benefits. The best approach is to do a little bit of everything. You'll look and feel great when you build a healthy heart for endurance, strong muscles for power, and develop flexibility to keep the body pliable.

Whether you are exercising to improve overall health or because you want to lose weight, research supports working out 1 hour a day, 5 days per week. The studies further revealed that those who exercised at least 5 hours a week were happiest with their bodies; while those that exercised less didn't get the results they were looking for.

Because it can be hard to devote a whole hour to a fitness routine it's fine to break it up throughout the day. Consider brief sessions of activity; for instance, if you can't fit in one 30-minute walk, try two 15 minute walks instead. Then add a strength building or flexibility training activity somewhere else in your day.

If you're not exercising at all right now I wouldn't suggest you jump to 5 hours a week right away; for many people that can be too much. The biggest reason people fail is because of the expectation that they can instantly make substantial changes. Instead ease into it. Focus on moving and exercising an hour or two a week and gradually challenge yourself to do a little more as time goes on. Remember the Kaizen Principle; your goals can be reached if practiced gradually, continuously, and constantly. The most important thing is to make a regular exercise program part of your lifestyle.

Many people will head straight to their local gym to get fitter, stronger and drop excess pounds. There you can typically chose from group classes, a variety of weight lifting options, an array of cardio machines, or hire a personal trainer. And while that's a great solution for some people, for others it can be a budget buster or too hard to fit into a daily routine. Fortunately, there are many other affordable, fun and interesting options available.

Joining a community center, a team, a local club, or taking a variety of classes that may be offered by your local parks & recreation department can be inexpensive as well as enjoyable. Walk or bicycle with friends, neighbors, or coworkers. Libraries offer a wide variety of options with DVD's to view and books to read before you decide to purchase. Technology offers app's for Smartphones, dedicated television channels and online programs for purchase at reasonable prices.

By mixing up your activities you are less likely to suffer from repetitive strain injuries. This type of injury often develops from repeated motions such as running, swimming, or hitting a tennis ball. It's important to give overused body parts a chance to rest and recover before putting them into action again. In the event you do get injured, choosing a different activity that doesn't burden the same part of the body will allow you to remain active and heal at the same time.

If you find yourself watching the clock and counting down the minutes while you're working out it may be time to switch up your routine. Beat boredom and prevent your workouts from getting stale by frequently trying new things. Attempt something new, venture into a dance class, try kickboxing, or sign up for martial arts lessons. Sometimes you have to start even when you think you're not ready. Be an asset to yourself by putting yourself out there; be open to showing up and trying things you've always wanted to do.

While making strides toward a healthier lifestyle it's common to reach plateaus. Your body gets use to the same activity and it will become very efficient; it's possible that you will burn fewer calories even when you're doing the same amount of work. The solution is to challenge yourself by incorporating new exercises and activities. Your body will have to work harder as it adjusts to the change of routine, therefore burning more calories when you work out. Remember that your diet is of major importance to reaching your health and fitness goals. The best abdominal exercise is 3 sets of stop eating so much crap!

Make a list of different types of exercise or activities you would enjoy or would like to learn more about.

CARDIOVASCULAR EXERCISE

Cardio, short for cardiovascular exercise, is a dreaded word for some, a passion for others. However you look at it, cardio is an essential part of every exercise program and should never be left out of your fitness plan.

Cardiovascular exercise is an aerobic activity, something which requires oxygen and enhances circulatory and respiratory efficiency. Cardiovascular exercise involves the movement of large muscle groups and requires a certain amount of endurance over a period of time, therefore increasing heart rate and blood circulation throughout the body. Examples include walking, jogging, and swimming; as well as the use of stationary machines like treadmills, ellipticals, and stair climbers. Group exercise classes such as spinning, dancing, and kickboxing are also great options for incorporating cardio into your workout.

Always start out at slowly; gradually building your strength and endurance. Be realistic and don't push yourself too hard, too fast. A comfortable balance between challenge and ease is important when selecting the energy level and type of exercise; always choose a suitable workout for you. Going overboard and running yourself into the ground serves no purpose and your chances for soreness, injury, and burnout increase.

The two basic ways to measure exercise intensity are perceived exertion and target heart rate.

PERCEIVED EXERTION

Perceived exertion is based on how hard the activity feels to you while you're doing it. It should fall into one of two categories; moderate intensity or vigorous intensity.

Moderate intensity feels reasonably hard.

- Your breathing quickens, but you're not out of breath.

- You develop a light sweat after 10 minutes of activity.

- You can carry on a conversation, but you can't sing.

Vigorous intensity feels demanding.

- Your breathing is deep and rapid.

- You develop a sweat after a few minutes of activity.

- You can only say a few words before pausing for a breath.

Studies show that your perceived exertion corresponds closely with your heart rate. If you think you're working hard, it's likely that your heart rate is elevated. So if you feel in tune with your body and your level of exertion, it's likely you will do fine using this simple method as a guide.

TARGET HEART RATE

Target heart rate is another method used to measure your level of intensity. To see how hard your heart is beating during physical activity you first have to figure out your maximum heart rate. Maximum heart rate is the number of times your heart should beat per minute while you're exercising.

To calculate maximum heart rate use the following formula:

220 – Your Age = Maximum Heart Rate

> Calculate your Maximum Heart Rate :
>
> *220 – Your Age = Maximum Heart Rate*

Once you have calculated your maximum heart rate, you can determine your desired target heart rate zone; the level at which your heart is being exercised and conditioned but not overworked.

Moderate intensity: 50 to 70 percent of your Maximum Heart Rate

Maximum Heart Rate x .50 = low end of moderate intensity

Maximum Heart Rate x .70 = high end of moderate intensity

> Calculate Moderate Intensity of your Maximum Heart Rate:
>
> *Maximum Heart Rate x .50 = low end of moderate intensity*
>
> *Maximum Heart Rate x .70 = high end of moderate intensity*

Vigorous intensity: 70 to 85 percent of your maximum heart rate

Maximum Heart Rate x .70 = low end of vigorous intensity

Maximum Heart Rate x .85 = high end of vigorous intensity

Calculate Vigorous Intensity of your Maximum Heart Rate:

Maximum Heart Rate x .70 = low end of vigorous intensity

Maximum Heart Rate x .85 = high end of vigorous intensity

If you embrace technology and want a more exact gauge of the numbers, a heart rate monitor will be a useful device for you. There are numerous choices at varying price points; a little bit of research online will help you decide which device is right for you.

Overall, you'll get the most from your workouts if you're exercising at the proper exercise intensity for your health and fitness goals. If you find that you're short of breath, physically uncomfortable or can't sustain your work out you're probably pushing yourself too hard. Listen to the cues your body is giving you; back off a bit and build your level of intensity more gradually. If you're strong and healthy and want more intensity, opt for the higher end of the zone. When you're not feeling you're working hard enough or your heart rate is too low, simply pick up the pace.

The Department of Health and Human Services recommends at least 150 minutes a week of moderate aerobic activity or 75 minutes a week of vigorous aerobic activity for healthy adults. Evenly spread throughout the week, cardio sessions should be at least 10 minutes long and can be divided throughout the day, such as three 10-minute walks. The key to receiving the benefits of aerobic activity is making it a part of your lifestyle.

If you find you must do an excessive amount of cardio throughout the week to burn off calories the answer is to direct your attention to your diet. While you can spend all day on the treadmill you will never outrun bad nutritional choices.

Regardless of your age, weight or fitness ability, aerobic exercise provides numerous benefits.

- Combined with a healthy diet, cardio supports weight loss and will help keep it off.

- Cardio will strengthen your heart. A stronger heart does not beat as fast and pumps blood more efficiently.

- Helping to keep your arteries clear by boosting your high-density lipoprotein (HDL), the good cholesterol, and lowering your low-density lipoprotein (LDL) the bad cholesterol, cardio results in less build-up of plaque in your arteries.

- Cardio reduces the risk of many conditions including high blood pressure, type 2 diabetes, depression, fatigue and anxiety. Weight-bearing exercise such as walking or step aerobics reduces the risk of osteoporosis

- Staying active as you age, cardio helps keep you strong and maintain your mobility, independence, and keeps your mind sharp. Studies reveal that 30 minutes of aerobic exercise 3 days a week reduces cognitive decline in older adults.

As your body becomes accustom to regular aerobic exercise, you'll see and feel your body get leaner, stronger and fitter. People who engage in a routine aerobic program live a longer and healthier life than those that don't exercise regularly.

If you have been inactive or have a chronic health condition you will want to visit your personal care physician before beginning any exercise plan. You should work closely with your health care provider to design and monitor a safe and effective plan for you. Remember slow and steady wins the race!

What types of aerobic activities are you interested in?

Decide upon a time and schedule an aerobic activity into your day.

Remember the Kaizen Principle; start slow and gradually increase the frequency working your way steadily, and consistently towards 150 minutes per week.

WEIGHT TRAINING

Who doesn't want to look good, feel better, and live a longer, stronger and healthier life?

Weight training, also commonly referred to as resistance or strength training, utilizes weights and the force of gravity for resistance to stress the skeletal muscles. Similar to the way aerobic conditioning strengthens your heart, weight training builds muscle strength and size, and contributes many functional benefits to the physique.

Participating in a weight training program will improve your body composition by decreasing fat mass and increasing lean body mass. It will boost your metabolism because your body needs to work harder to maintain muscle over fat, therefore burning more calories throughout the day.

As you age, you naturally lose bone mass. Just as your muscles will build and grow from the stress of weightlifting, so will your bones. When your bones perceive stress, your bodies response is to build more bone, therefore increasing bone density and lowering the risk of osteoporosis.

By raising your level of endorphins, the natural opiates produced by the brain, weight training has been shown to increase energy, improve mood, and has been proven to be a great antidepressant.

Studies show that weight training plays a significant role in reducing the risk of many chronic conditions including, arthritis, heart disease, diabetes, high blood pressure and back pain.

If that isn't enough to convince you, weight training will benefit sleep quality, sharpen focus, and increase stamina; improving your overall quality of life.

A workout at your local gym does not have to be an intimidating experience nor does a weight training program need to be a daunting endeavor. When looking around any gym it's likely you will be overwhelmed by the multitude of machines and equipment. What is all this equipment and how does it work? Even the jargon seems like a foreign language. If you are ready to begin an exercise program and require instruction and support, hiring a personal trainer can provide you the guidance you need to reach your fitness goals.

Based on a comprehensive personal fitness evaluation and individual goals, a personal trainer will develop the most effective routine for you. Beginners will also benefit from instruction on how to perform specific exercises, as well as the proper and safe use of equipment.

With today's hectic lifestyles no one has time to waste on ineffective routines and sticking to a program can sometimes prove to be difficult. By scheduling regular appointments with a trainer, you can maximize your time and eliminate excuses for not working out. Personalized programs that meet your needs and level of fitness will move you forward much more quickly, safely, and efficiently than working out on your own.

Personal trainers provide their expertise to help you achieve your health and fitness goals. They are there to observe and provide you with feedback, assist and adjust you through your workout, raise your confidence, and motivate you to take your workout to the next level.

Don't limit yourself to thinking that a gym membership is the only way to do strength training; it can easily and affordably be done in the privacy and convenience of your home. Remember your local library offers many choices in the form of instructional DVD's and books to view. There are a wide variety of health and fitness magazines, Smartphone app's, and television programming choices to keep your routine interesting and challenging.

Equipment isn't necessary to target and build muscle; many exercises can be performed using your own bodyweight. Otherwise, reasonably priced and readily available resistance bands, exercise balls, and free weights can be used to enhance your weight training program.

As you can see weight training offers a multitude of health benefits. You don't need to dedicate several hours a day lifting to reap the rewards. Two to three sessions a week lasting just 20 to 30 minutes are sufficient for most people and the results are quickly accomplished.

Expect to see noticeable changes in just a few weeks when you combine your training with a positive attitude and healthy food choices. You can live at the gym, but if you don't eat right you are wasting your time. Your diet will always be number one. If you don't eat healthy food in the proper amount no amount of time spent in the gym will help you reach your fitness goals. Those ab's you want, they're made in the kitchen. You cannot out train a bad diet!

Explore a variety of weight training programs by viewing DVD's, Smartphone App's, online videos, or by attending classes or hiring a personal trainer. When you find a form of exercise that you enjoy you are more likely to incorporate it into a routine program.

What are some strength training methods you would like to try?

Where can you schedule 2 to 3, 20 to 30-minute weight training sessions per week into your schedule?

Lifting Weights = More Muscle, More Muscle = Greater Metabolism, Greater Metabolism = Weight Loss!

FLEXIBILITY AND BALANCE

As a master yoga instructor I have led a multitude of students through thousands of hours of yoga classes. So it is with certainty I can say that flexibility and balance are two of the most overlooked and under practiced components to a well-rounded fitness regimen.

Many people will work hard running on a treadmill or lifting weights but be tempted to skip exercises that promote mobility and stability in favor of those that they feel offer a bigger bang for their buck.

Both flexibility and balance exercises are important and relevant especially after doing weight training and cardiovascular exercise. Stretching slowly and deliberately plays a clear role in your overall level of fitness and body function. It increases your range of motion and conditions the muscles helping to keep them limber and prevent cramping.

A regular yoga practice offers many vital physical and mental health benefits. Some physical gains, like increased energy and circulation, better posture and muscle control, and improved balance and coordination are noticeably evident. Other mental health benefits, such as a reduction in stress levels, anxiety, and irritability; improved focus, creativity, and mood; elevated self-esteem, self-confidence, and self-control, may be subtle but they are just as effective.

When you add up the benefits it's easy to see why yoga has become an increasingly popular and mainstream practice in the United States. Experts agree that yoga has a rejuvenating effect on the body, contributes to a heightened sense of well-being, and is a great compliment to any exercise program.

If you are just beginning a yoga practice you will find that you have many options to choose from. With so many styles of yoga and types of classes being offered, selecting the best yoga class for you will be a personal choice. Classes that are labeled beginner, basic, or gentle are generally suitable for all.

To get the most benefit and enjoyment it's important to try different classes and instructors and see what suits your fitness levels and goals. Are the instructions understandable making it easy to follow? Is the class manageable yet challenging? Do you feel comfortable and are you having fun? Give it a little time and let your personal experience guide you.

Every teacher will have their own unique style based on their personality, fitness background, and with whom they have trained. Look for someone who you can relate to; someone who inspires you and encourages you, someone who has an understanding and compassion for where you are in your journey to well-being. A genuine teacher does not seek to impress you with their greatness, but impress upon you that you possess the skills to discover your own.

If you don't have the time or money to go to a studio or a gym to take a yoga class it can easily be done in the comfort and privacy of your home. Try some different yoga styles by viewing DVD's you can check out from your local library, watch one of the many shows on TV, or search online for free videos to follow along with.

Make an effort to incorporate a yoga practice into your exercise program two or three times a week, for at least 30 minutes to an hour. Don't let your lack of time or unrealistic goals become an obstacle. If all you can devote is 20 minutes, that's fine too. Do what you can and don't worry about it, just start somewhere. It's likely that your inclination to practice will increase and you will find yourself easily integrating this beneficial modality into your everyday life. A regular yoga practice will be the foundation needed to boost your energy and guide you to more healthful daily habits. Your present situation is not your final destination; you are a work in progress!

Where in your schedule can you devote at least 20 to 30 minutes, 2 or 3 times a week to a simple yoga practice?

Where are you most comfortable and most likely to practice yoga?

If you answered in the privacy of your home, look for videos online, programs on television, or check out one of the many DVD's available. If you want more instruction and structure try joining a health club that offers yoga classes or join a studio for more hands on instruction.

BEYOND PHYSICAL FITNESS

People generally think of exercise in terms of physical health but do not consider its effect on mental health. Much research has been done in the last decade that reveals exercise to be a powerful tool in the optimization of brain function. These studies continually show that your body and your brain are connected. The more you work at getting your body in shape the more adaptable and responsive your brain becomes both cognitively and psychologically.

With physical activity, senses become heightened having a positive impact on your levels of energy and passion, interest and motivation, mood and self-esteem. The simple act of being in motion has been shown to promote the belief that you can reach your goals and bring them to successful completion.

Regular exercise is essential and packs a powerful punch when it comes to brain health and learning. From keeping your brain sharp by improving its potential to process new information, to deepening attention span and focus, and developing a greater capacity for memory and cognitive efficiency, activity helps to keep your neurons firing.

Opt for workouts that keep you engaged and attentive; it is essential that you change up your routine and include activities that foster a challenge. Maintaining an active lifestyle is a crucial and vital investment in your future well-being.

MEDITATION

In the words of world renowned doctor and alternative medicine advocate Deepak Chopra, "Meditation is not a way of making your mind quiet. It is a way of entering into the quiet that is already there buried under the 50,000 thoughts that the average person thinks every day."

Comparable to the way that fitness is an approach to training the body, meditation is an approach to training the mind. Mindful meditation is a practice of paying careful attention to what is happening moment-by-moment and believing there is no right or wrong way to feel at any given time. It is a discipline of purposely engaging your attention on your thoughts, feelings, senses and the surrounding environment and accepting it without judgment.

Don't be concerned that you aren't able to sit the full lotus position for hours in a saffron robe and pretend you're a statue with an empty mind. There are several distinct meditative practices that require different mental skills. Do a little research online; there are many videos and downloads available to guide you through a meditation practice.

This simple mindful meditation exercise is an excellent introduction for beginners.

- Designate a place that is quiet and comfortable.

- Set a timer. Remember the Kaizen Principle; perhaps begin with 3 minutes and gradually increase the length of time to suit your needs and abilities.

- Sit or lie comfortably.

- Close your eyes.

- Breathe naturally. Don't make any effort to control your breath.

- Focus your attention on the breath and the rise and fall of the body with each inhalation and exhalation.

- When your mind wanders, let go of the thought and bring your awareness back to your breath.

If you find it difficult to sit quietly and meditate in the traditional manner a productive alternative is moving meditation. A moving meditation allows you to break free from the conventional rules and constriction of a seated practice; turning any form of conscious movement into meditation. Many activities can be used as an opportunity to cultivate peace and serenity; Yoga, Tai Chi, walking, dancing and playing a musical instrument are all forms of a moving meditation.

The benefits of meditation are many and will be unique to the individual. Perhaps Buddha said it best when asked, "What have you gained from meditation?" He replied "Nothing. However, let me tell you what I have lost; anger, anxiety, depression, insecurity, fear of old age and death."

SLEEP AND WEIGHT LOSS

Nearly everyone knows that to trim down and lose weight they should decrease food intake and increase exercise. Another critical, yet lesser known component to weight control is sleep deprivation. Sleep is like Miracle–Gro for the brain. The average person requires 7 to 9 hours of sleep each night; for many not getting enough sleep is a routine experience.

There is compelling scientific evidence that insufficient sleep promotes hunger and appetite, which can cause overeating resulting in weight gain. The mere act of sleeping doesn't mean you will lose weight. If you are not getting enough sleep or a good quality of sleep your metabolism will suffer the consequences by not running efficiently.

Your ability to lose weight has a lot to do two key hormones, leptin and ghrelin. Not getting enough hours of quality sleep will cause leptin levels to plunge and ghrelin levels to rise. Leptin is the hormone that tells your brain that your stomach is full and to stop eating. Ghrelin is the hormone that stimulates your appetite making it more difficult to resist eating. Therefore, less leptin and more ghrelin add up to weight gain.

Then there is the spike in cortisol; a hormone which is released when you are under stress and is responsible for regulating your appetite. The *Journal of the American Medical Association* suggests that a loss of sleep can make you feel hungrier as the production of cortisol increases causing you to overeat and store excess body fat. Furthermore, sleep loss can influence and disturb the body's metabolism, which will hamper your ability to lose weight.

It's important to make sure that you get the rest your body needs. When your body is fully rested and you are getting the deep sleep you require, your hormones will work together and support your overall health and fitness goals.

EXERCISING AS A FAMILY

The American Heart Association reports that approximately one in three American children and teens are overweight or obese; more than tripling in number from 1971 to 2011. Childhood obesity is now the number one health related issue concerning parents in the United States, surpassing drug abuse and smoking.

Childhood obesity is causing a broad range of health problems including high blood pressure, Type 2 diabetes and elevated blood cholesterol levels. As well there are psychological effects; obese children are more prone to low self-esteem, negative body image, and depression.

Possibly the most sobering statement with respect to the severity of the childhood obesity epidemic came from former Surgeon General Richard Carmona, "Because of the increasing rates of obesity, unhealthy eating habits and physical inactivity, we may see the first generation that will be less healthy and have a shorter life expectancy than their parents."

As a parent it is imperative to cultivate a culture of wellness as a family; your children's attitudes and actions will model your behavior. Spending time together exercising is a great way to set a good example and help your children develop positive habits at a young age.

Find fun activities to participate in by contacting your local recreation centers, civic organizations or clubs that are of interest to you. Exercising as a family is beneficial for you and for them; it will build and enhance social skills, self-esteem, and self-confidence, and deepen your relationship with your children. It is in this environment that children learn healthy habits are a positive way of life. Get off of the sofa and get away from the screens, get up and get moving!

We all must travel the distance of a lifetime in this body. If we don't care for it how can we reach our goals?

—Swami Kripalu

IN HEALTH

- Excuses get you nowhere, you're going to have to dig deep. Identify the issues you are facing and give all of your spirit and energy to finding a solution. Your future is wide open and you have the power to create it by what you choose to do.

- Stepping out of your comfort zone to begin an exercise program can be scary. Trust me when I tell you that doubting yourself will kill more of your dreams than failure ever will. Exercise does not need to be a chore. Stay fit by choosing activities that you love.

- Consulting your primary care physician is of importance when starting any type of exercise program. Take time to discuss the different modalities including cardiovascular exercise, weight training, and flexibility/balance. While the Department of Health and Human Services offers guidelines they don't know you. It is imperative that you and your doctor determine a sensible and safe starting point for you.

- Increase your level of fitness by incorporating activities that enhance your brain function and mental wellness. Yoga and meditation have an artful, clever way of circumventing the mental patterns that cause stress and anxiety. The conscious brain can think only one thought at a time. Move toward a bigger, brighter future of your choosing by reflecting on positive thoughts.

- There is conclusive evidence that the quality of your sleep has a significant impact on hunger and appetite. Lower metabolism and out of control hormones will cause your body to run inefficiently. Be aware of your sleep patterns by recording them in your journal.

- Childhood obesity is rampant. It is slowly spiraling out of control and continuing to rise at an alarming rate. Spend time being active with your children and create healthy habits that will last a lifetime.

Download and print your free companion workbook at www.judymolinaro.com/p/workbook.

Final Thoughts

Start from where you are with what you've got and go where it is you want to go.

Zig Ziglar

Now that you've read the book and understand the basic principles for healthy living it's time for you to do the hard work. Please don't be afraid of trying. Take it one step at a time; remember every journey has to begin somewhere. Keep in mind that no matter how you feel, in order to reach your goals, you must get up, show up, and never, ever give up!

Being consistent will be the key to your success. Follow the principles you have learned on a daily basis; eat well and exercise regularly. The changes will not happen overnight; at times you will be overwhelmed and may be discouraged. Please put one foot in front of the other; keep on keeping on. You are building the foundation for living a healthy lifestyle 24/7; you must trust the process.

Keeping up with journaling, weighing in, measuring, and assessing your progress as you go will be critical to your success. These periodic practices will keep you on track by giving you regular feedback and help you detect small changes both positive and negative. It's easy to get lazy and think "I've got this"; always be mindful of your choices and the habits you are creating.

Even when you have reached your goals you must stay on track on a daily basis. In order to maintain your new level of fitness you must be aware of the inclination to slip back into old routines. Don't look back, you're not going that way; look at your results and rely on them to motivate you.

Find a strong network of people who support your endeavors, they will be critical to realizing your goals. This group may be made up of friends, family members, co-workers, fitness professionals, social groups etc. It has been said that we are a combination of the five people we are closest to and that their influence can be considerable.

If you interact with people who eat well and exercise chances are you will too. Without even knowing it their behaviors, actions and habits will teach you things about grocery shopping, eating out and food preparation. The takeaway is to always surround yourself with like-minded people as they will be a large part of your formula for success.

Be mindful of the food and emotional triggers that can cause you to fall off of your eating plan. Susceptibility to these triggers will vary among individuals; they can be set off by any number of things, and they are likely to happen. For some it might be walking into a movie theater or going to a buffet restaurant, for others it will be attending a party, or a sporting event. Certain emotions can also set off these triggers; issues like stress at work, money concerns, or a sad event can easily and quickly initiate overeating. The bottom line is when it happens, recognize it and have positive strategies in place to cope with the situation.

Your accomplishments will require more than just your adherence to a regimen of eating and exercise. Its foundation lies in your attitude and having a clear understanding of who you are; mind, body and spirit.

Success is what you say it is; don't let others define it for you. You are a priority. You are your own author. What is the story you want to write about yourself? It's time to dust off your dreams and sweep your own ass off of your feet!

The next time someone asks what you weigh tell them a hundred and sexy!

About the Author

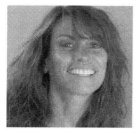

As a personal development and wellness coach Judy Molinaro empowers people seeking breakthroughs in their private and professional lives to develop high performance habits. Attentive and insightful to her client's needs she is known to lead with a firm hand and a compassionate heart. A master instructor who instills confidence and awareness, her lessons are skillfully crafted and easy to follow making her a sought after expert in her field.

Through her Fit You Wellness Solutions program she forms partnerships with clients and presents her decades of experience in the fitness industry as a workshop facilitator and speaker. She helps people find their fire, re-ignite their passion, and lead extraordinary, fully charged lives.

She has expanded her performance programs to include BeneFit You Wellness Solutions collaborating with non-profit agencies to create unique fundraising campaigns. Deepening the connection of companies to their community and rallying civic minded people around causes of social good she endeavors to leave the world a little better place than she found it.

An animal welfare advocate, foster mom to dozens of abandoned pets and lover of all things wild, Judy is a founding member of Concerned Citizens for Animal Welfare a non-profit corporation dedicated to reducing animal overpopulation. A New England native, she lives in Ormond Beach, Florida with her cats Sissy and LuLu.

We make a living by what we get, but we make a life by what we give.

—Winston Churchill

Visit Judy:
www.judymolinaro.com
www.facebook.com/fityouwellness

FOR MORE INFORMATION

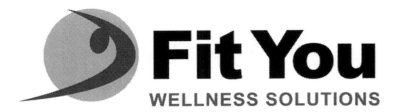

Cultivating a High Energy Workforce

What would it be like to surrender to the belief that a few simple habits practiced daily will lead to an increase in performance and productivity in your personal and professional life?

As a speaker and workshop facilitator Judy Molinaro shares her experience and expertise in the wellness industry with seminar attendees. Her creative, spirited style keeps the audience involved and entertained. Whether for an hour, a day, or expanded with progressive coaching, her Fit You Wellness Solutions© programs are a catalyst for the evolution and growth of your business.

Through her interactive presentations she introduces an integrated approach to wellness; the linking together of personal responsibility, self-education, and physical development to make sustainable transformations. Putting fresh ideas into action, Judy's workshops are custom designed to meet your needs and targeted to your team's goals.

Hire performance consultant Judy Molinaro to re-ignite wellness and empower your team!

For booking information and availability contact:
judy@judymolinaro.com or 386.871.0582

Visit Judy:
www.judymolinaro.com
www.facebook.com/fityouwellness

Bene **Fit You**

Fundraising for Social Cause

- Is your business looking for ways to connect and give back to the community?

- Is your charitable organization seeking original ideas to raise funds and awareness for your cause?

Through BeneFit You Wellness Solutions© Judy combines her knowledge in personal development, nutrition, and fitness with her passion to serve others leaving the world a little better place than she found it. She is excited to collaborate with corporate partners, philanthropists, and charitable organizations who share a vision in social initiatives that strengthen their communities.

Joining forces to build distinctive workshops and fundraising campaigns, Judy strives to deepen the connection of companies to their community by rallying civic minded people around causes of social good. Each presentation is unique and creatively linked to the project based on your vision and targeted outcome.

Contact Judy Molinaro to help you make your charity event a resounding success.

For booking information and availability contact:
judy@judymolinaro.com or 386.871.0582

Visit Judy:
www.judymolinaro.com
www.facebook.com/fityouwellness

Acknowledgements

Where does one begin when saying thank you? When is enough, enough when so many people have played a significant role in your journey? What does it take to capture and convey the essence of an individual's effect on your life in a few sentences? How does one cull through the nostalgia and extract what is buried deep inside a lifetime of memories?

It is with a genuine heart, I acknowledge and thank those that have supported me in my efforts to see this book to completion.

Pam Carrier, who would have thought that all those hours spent at FHS in classroom G-138 would have brought us here? Not only are you a valued childhood friend, you are a mentor and a cheerleader. Your artistic ability, ingenuity, and professional guidance have taken this project to a place beyond my wildest dreams. Kevin Snyder, thank you for helping me set the course from the start, lending an ear, and fitting me into your busy and exciting schedule. John Sannicandro it is my good fortune that you are the kind of guy who, when asked will help a friend. Thank you for offering your thoughts and sharing your enthusiasm for this project. Sandy Kangas your kind words and vote of confidence for this book meant more than you could imagine. Kathy Hardy you are an exquisite hand model, a fun driveway sitter and generous sharer of chocolate and chit chat. Paul Vicario, we've come a long way from our days spent together at SMS. Thank you for sharing your time and creative talents; your generosity is greatly appreciated. Bob Baumer your encouragement, enthusiasm, and professional guidance brought this project to a whole new level. Lucky me that our paths crossed and that I call you friend. And finally, to the boy next door, a one-time life-long friend gone ghost. Thank you for opening my eyes and showing me what I'm capable of when put to the test. It's because of you that I am marching to the beat of a different drummer.

NOTES

NOTES

NOTES

NOTES

NOTES

NOTES

NOTES

NOTES

NOTES

NOTES

NOTES

Made in the USA
Las Vegas, NV
28 November 2020